# New Research in Nursing - Education and Practice

*Edited by Victor Chaban*

Published in London, United Kingdom

New Research in Nursing - Education and Practice
http://dx.doi.org/10.5772/intechopen.108428
Edited by Victor Chaban

Contributors
Chandra Rekha Makanjee, Razzagh Rahimpoor, Jia Guo, Ehsan Garosi, Delgersuren Gelegjamts, Khulan Gaalan, Batbagana Burenerdene, Priscilla Yeye Adumoah Attafuah, Cecilia Eliason, Ninon P. Amertil, Sarah A. Balcom, Doris Y.P. Leung, Helen Y.L. Chan, Patrick K.C. Chiu, Raymond S.K. Lo, Geeta Parwanda, Serly Sani Mahoklory, Ferdinandus Suban Hoda, Marvin J. Gordon, Ka-Huen Yip, Tze-Wing Wong, Yuk Chiu Yip, Wai-King Tsui, R.N. Hiroko Shimizu



First published in London, United Kingdom, 2023 by IntechOpen
IntechOpen is the global imprint of INTECHOPEN LIMITED, registered in England and Wales, registration number: 11086078, 5 Princes Gate Court, London, SW7 2QJ, United Kingdom

British Library Cataloguing-in-Publication Data
A catalogue record for this book is available from the British Library

Additional hard and PDF copies can be obtained from orders@intechopen.com

New Research in Nursing - Education and Practice
Edited by Victor Chaban
p. cm.
Print ISBN 978-1-80355-081-7
Online ISBN 978-1-80355-082-4
eBook (PDF) ISBN 978-1-80355-083-1

For EU product safety concerns:
IN TECH d.o.o., Prolaz Marije Krucifikse Kozulić 3, 51000 Rijeka, Croatia,
info@intechopen.com or visit our website at intechopen.com.

# Meet the editor

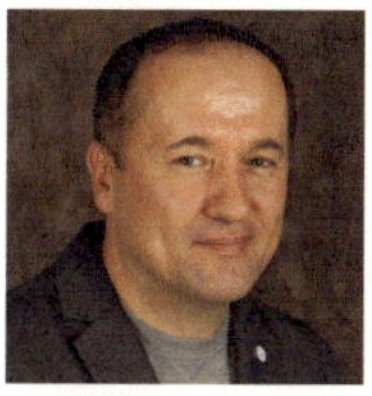

Dr. Victor V. Chaban is chairman of the Department of Biomedical Science Education and Professor of Medicine with dual appointments at the Charles R. Drew University of Medicine and Science (CDU), California, USA, and the University of California Los Angeles (UCLA). Dr. Chaban completed his post-doctoral training in neuroscience at UCLA and graduate studies in clinical research at CDU. He is serving at the US National Institutes of Health (NIH) and several international study sections and holds US patents. Dr. Chaban is editor-in-chief for the *International Journal of Research in Nursing* and a member of several journal editorial boards. He is an author/editor of five books.

# Contents

# Preface

Nursing plays a vital role in healthcare systems worldwide. It encompasses not only research and education but also compassionate care for patients and communities, promotion of health, and advocacy for overall well-being. Today, understanding and meeting patient concerns is as important as performing therapeutic interventions in the evidence-based practice of healthcare delivery.

New Research in Nursing – Education and Practice provides an overview of current nursing experience in novel clinical interventions. The authors are a group of international experts with expertise in the various clinical aspects upon which the practice components of nursing care are based. We hope that many of the therapeutic advances described in this book will allow nurses and other healthcare professionals to use best practices to improve healthcare outcomes.

This book contains a diverse range of research studies that address critical areas within nursing. These studies delve into various dimensions of nursing education and interdisciplinary collaboration. The authors have examined their findings, employing different methodologies and best practices, and I wish to express my sincere thanks to all who have contributed to this book. Each chapter focuses on specific nursing interventions and novel strategies investigating the impact of technological advancements on nursing practice and nursing education.

In Chapter 1, R.N. Hiroko Shimizu presents an evaluation of nurses' attitudes toward elderly care. In Chapter 2, Geeta Parwanda discusses reflective approaches in nursing education and clinical practice. In Chapter 3, Sarah A. Balcom focuses on advanced practice nursing in Canada. In Chapter 4, Jia Guo demonstrates the application of operation research to health care. In Chapter 5, Chandra Rekha Makanjee discusses nurse practitioners' "insider" and "outsider" roles and responsibilities enabling quality managed delivery of medical imaging services. In Chapters 6 and 7, Marvin J. Gordon and Delgersuren Gelegjamts et al., discuss palliative care. In Chapter 8, Ka-Huen Yip et al., discuss advances in burn care in Hong Kong. In Chapter 9, Razzagh Rahimpoor presents the physiological and physical effects of sleep disorders. In Chapter 10, Doris Y.P. Leung shows the effects of video-supported, nurse-led advance care planning for older adults with frailty. In Chapter 11, Priscilla Yeye Adumoah Attafuah et al., talk about reconceptualising geriatric care in sub-Saharan Africa. In Chapter 12, Serly Sani Mahoklory and Ferdinandus Suban Hoda discuss the effect of cromotherapy on decreased blood pressure in patients in Indonesia. Finally, in Chapter 13, Ehsan Garosi presents nurse work system organization through the lens of macro ergonomics.

While it is very difficult to provide an overview of all aspects of nursing, we hope that this book will be a valuable resource not only for nurses but also for other clinicians, students, and patients seeking insights into new therapies and clinical practices. In this book, you can navigate the evolving landscape of nursing practice that addresses the challenges and opportunities faced by healthcare providers worldwide. I encourage readers from other backgrounds to read this collection of excellent publications as a source of inspiration for critical thinking and new ideas in education and clinical investigation. Finally, I would like to acknowledge the publishing team who have worked tirelessly to bring this collection to the audience.

**Victor Chaban, Ph.D., MSCR**
Chairman and Professor,
Department of Biomedical Science Education,
Charles R. Drew University of Medicine and Science,

Professor,
Department of Medicine
University of California,
Los Angeles, USA

Chapter 1

# Evaluation and Cultural Influence of Nurses' Attitudes toward Elderly Care

*R.N. Hiroko Shimizu*


## Abstract

The eldery population among the 38 countries of the Organization for Economic Co-operation and Development; thus, nurses have many opportunities to care for the elderly. The elderly are more likely to suffer from diseases, such as geriatric syndrome and sarcopenia, in addition to frailty. Medical personnel is reported to have a protective attitude, but the problems of nurses' dialog attitudes include confusion, concern, prejudice, and difficulty in dialog with patients with critical illnesses. Therefore, we had developed the scale to evaluate the negative aspects of nurses' interactive attitudes toward the elderly. The validity and reliability for the scale of the 15-item and 7-law methods were determined. A comparison of the dialog orientation scales of nurses and nursing students revealed that nurses are more positive as they gain more experience. Additionally, nurses were more negative about age discrimination in dialog and the difficulty of dialog with seriously injured people than caregivers because nurses care for more severely ill elderly. Moreover, we implemented a program to conduct dialog training with the elderly from the stage of nursing students, which revealed a clear effect.


**Keywords:** elderly care, nurse, prejudiced attitude, cognitive bias, Japan

## 1. Introduction

This chapter provides research-based insights for improving the quality of care for the elderly, particularly within New Research in Nursing – Education and Practice. The important keywords are "successful aging" and "age discrimination." Focusing on age discrimination, especially cognitive distortions in caregivers, is necessary for the elderly to achieve happy aging.

Before the 1980s, aging was viewed as a period of increasing physical and mental frailty. However, this viewpoint has clearly changed since the early 1990s and has been influenced by the notion of "successful aging" advocated by Rowe and Kahn [1]. As expressed in the terminal decline model proposed by psychologists, crystalized intelligence continues to function until just before death, and older people are capable of contributing to society, which should be considered a desirable objective [2]. Nurses involved in healthcare with older people should understand the characteristics of aging and be free of cognitive bias when treating older people [3]. Ageism discrimination is one of these cognitive biases.

Ageism refers to cognitive bias toward older people and is a specific form of discrimination, such as racism and sexism. Specifically, Butler [4] defined ageism as "a process of systematic stereotyping and discrimination against people because they are old." This type of bias, which results from cultural and social influences [5], is distinctive for each country and ethnic group. This may be a specific problem in Japan, with Palmore [5] observing that the general Japanese population holds feelings of respect and contempt for older people. Indeed, it can be difficult to correct through education.

In February and March 2004, the Japanese Cabinet Office performed the "Survey on Public Attitudes to Aging," which used the Fraboni Scale of Ageism (FSA) to evaluate cognitive bias against older people among 6000 Japanese respondents aged ≥20 years. Respondents who were older males living in major cities or prone to illness expressed strong feelings of avoidance and rejection toward older people. People form views about others beginning from their childhood who influenced by one's family and community. Another research in Japan indicated that views toward older people are positive in elementary school but less positive in junior high school and high school. Children frequently consider older people to be physically weak [6]. In other words, cognition changes negatively with the time affected. Therefore, Japanese culture and social influences may enhance the prejudice against older people.

## 2. Increasing number of elderly people in the population

### 2.1 Japanese average life expectancy and high aging rate

Japan's Ministry of Health, Labor, and Welfare reported a Japanese population of 122,780,487 as of October 1, 2021, following a year-on-year downward trend since 2007.

The population aged ≥65 years in Japan accounted for 36,214,000, with an increase of 188,000 from the previous year, having the highest ratio of 28.9%.

The population aged ≥75 years accounted for 18,674,000, with an increase of 72,000 from the previous year, having the highest ratio of 14.9%. The total ratio of elderly people aged ≥65 years was 42.38 in the population [7]. Hence, one in two or three Japanese people is an elderly person.

The average life expectancy of the Japanese was the highest ever in 2020. The most recent average life expectancy increased by 0.09 and 0.14 years in 2021, with an average of 81.47 and 87.57 years for males and females, respectively. The difference in life expectancy between males and females was 6.10 years, which decreased by 0.05 years from the previous year. Therefore, the life expectancy of males has relatively increased [8].

These results reveal that the elderly who need care mainly consists of people in their 80s.

Deaths in 2021 increased to a postwar high of 1,439,856 (increased by 67,101 from 1,372,755 in 2020).

The number of deaths from malignant neoplasm (tumor) was 381,505 (26.5% of the total number of deaths), and the mortality rate (per 100,000 population) of 310.7 ranked first place, followed by heart disease (14.9%, 174.9), senility (10.6%, 123.8), cerebrovascular disease, and pneumonia, in order.

The number of deaths due to coronavirus disease 2019 (COVID-19) was 16,766.

These diseases are among the leading causes of death in the elderly. The majority of Japanese elderly patients in end-of-life care have chronic diseases, such as cancer, heart disease, cerebrovascular disease, and pneumonia, in addition to senility. However, the number of patients following an acute turning point due to COVID-19 infection has increased since 2020. Thus, many patients with chronic diseases require a long treatment period, and they have a long relationship with nurses. Particularly, nurses' attitudes possibly affect the quality of nurses.

### 2.2 International comparison of the aging rate

The Organization for Economic Co-operation and Development (OECD) is an international organization with 38 developed countries, mainly European countries, including Japan and the United States. The OECD database predicted Japan to have the fastest-aging population worldwide by 2021. From this point of view, Japan's approach to measures and care for the elderly may set a precedent for other countries [9, 10].

Countries with high aging rates often have low birth rates and total fertility rates. Therefore, an economic guarantee for care is important because it is accompanied by a decreased working-age population. The economic precedent for elderly care in Japan is the Long-Term Care Insurance Law [8].

The aging rate in Japan was at the bottom, middle, and highest in the 1980s, the 1990s, and 2005, respectively, compared to that of other developed countries. This high level is expected to be maintained in the future.

Comparing the number of years required for the aging rate to reach 14%, 126 years in France, 85 years in Sweden, 72 years in the United States, and 126 years in Sweden, compared to relatively short periods of 46 years for the United Kingdom and 40 years for Germany, Japan exceeded 7% in 1970 and reached 14% in 1994, 24 years later.

Conversely, some Asian countries, such as South Korea in 2018 and Singapore in 2017, are expected to have a faster aging speed than Japan [11].

## 3. Geriatric medicine and characteristics

### 3.1 Physical changes in the elderly

Many elderly people have physical decline or frailty, with age. Frailty in the elderly not only reduces the quality of life but also carries the risk of various complications.

A research group of the Ministry of Health, Labor, and Welfare in Japan defined frailty as "mental and physical vitality (motor function, cognitive function, etc.) decreases with aging, and life functions are impaired due to the effects of multiple chronic diseases, etc., and is a state in which physical and mental vulnerability has emerged." Conversely, frailty is considered a state in which maintaining and improving living functions are possible through appropriate intervention and support, and appropriate intervention by nurses is required [12].

We calculated the frailty rate of Japanese elderly people through a panel survey, because Japan has the highest aging rate worldwide. The results showed that the rate of frailty was 8.7% among all elderly people. Hence, approximately 11.3 million elderly people in Japan require appropriate intervention and support. They are the target of nursing care, including the elderly living at home, because not all of these are inpatients. Therefore, nurses should increase their knowledge of the elderly to improve the effectiveness of care because the elderly are important subjects of care [13].

Japan will have 960,000 nurses, including registered and associate nurses, by 2021, with at least one frail elderly person for every nurse. Japanese nurses work in a wide variety of fields, including clinics, healthcare facilities for the elderly, welfare facilities for the elderly, and home-visit nursing, in addition to hospitals. The attitude that nurses take toward the elderly is hypothesized to affect the quality of intervention and support because nurses provide face-to-face life support.

### 3.2 Diseases of the elderly

The elderly have various diseases, but these diseases are very different from patients at other developmental stages, such as adults and children. Diseases that are common among the elderly in Japan include geriatric syndrome, sarcopenia/frailty, locomotive syndrome, dementia, cancer, infectious diseases, aspiration lung disease, pneumonia, diabetes and its complications, and hypertension. A geriatric syndrome is a general term for symptoms and signs that are often seen in the elderly with aging and require a medical examination, care, and nursing care. The geriatric syndrome has >50 items of symptoms and signs and is characterized by having multiple symptoms; thus, patients are required to visit multiple clinical departments and hospitals. Physiological aging and pathological aging coexist in geriatric syndrome; thus, factors and effects for recovery should be correctly evaluated. Diseases associated with the geriatric syndrome include hormonal depletion and lacunar infarction. Hormones are associated with the decline of aging and may be treated with hormone replacement therapy [14, 15].

### 3.3 Points to note in elderly care

Elderly people experience a decline in activities of daily living (ADLs) when they are ill as typified by the geriatric syndrome. The risk factors that double this decline in ADL are cognition, sensory fatigue, falls, depression, and female sex. Cerebrovascular accidents increase the risk fivefold. Moderate aerobic exercise and interactive communication are necessary to avoid these.

Sarcopenia, which is common in the elderly, refers to the loss of muscle mass and muscle strength due to aging, and in October 2016, "sarcopenia" was registered in the International Classification of Diseases and is now positioned as a disease. Sarcopenia affects ADLs, such as walking and standing, requires care, and is prone to falls. Approximately 15% of the elderly aged ≥65 in Japan are considered affected by sarcopenia. As of 2019, the elderly population is estimated to be 35.89 million; hence, approximately 5 million elderly people are likely to have sarcopenia. However, exercise and nutrition are expected to improve muscles even after 70 years old; thus, so exercise and nutrition are important factors in the care of the elderly [13].

## 4. Attitudes of nurses in geriatric nursing

The elderly have more opportunities to receive nursing care due to symptoms and disabilities caused by aging and illness. The caregiver's dialog and attitude greatly affect the willingness of the elderly to recover and rehabilitate.

An example is based on Bandura's theory of social learning. According to his theory, the factors that influence the patient's behavior are not only the family members but also the nurse's emotional arousal and model behavior presentation, which affect the outcome of care. Numerous studies were conducted on this issue of nurses' care attitudes in nursing the elderly, and nurses' knowledge and attitudes are considered important for high-quality care.

### 4.1 Characteristics and problems of nurses' attitudes toward the elderly

The author focused on the dialog between nurses and the elderly and clarified the problems and characteristics of dialog.

The research method was a questionnaire survey using the indwelling method for 833 nursing students. The questionnaire consisted of 43 items whose content validity was confirmed. The evaluation scale was a 7-point scale ranging from "strongly agree" to "strongly disagree." Exploratory factor analysis and multidimensional scaling, which are analysis methods by IBM's SPSS, were used for analysis. As a result, four factors were extracted as characteristics of conversations between nursing students and the elderly. The factors were ``confused about involvement," ``concern about involvement," ``prejudice about involvement," and ``difficulty about involvement." These factors represented the attitudes of nursing students influenced by emotions such as anxiety toward the elderly, and the values of nursing students toward the elderly. Also, the characteristic of dialog was the concept placed on the two axes of cognition and attitude. The problem of attitudes of nurses found here can be an important evaluation index for education of nurses.

### 4.2 Evaluation of factors affecting nurses' attitudes

Disability due to aging has been the most emphasized problem among the target elderly people. For example, ADL indicators [16], dementia-related memory ability evaluation [17], and hearing ability in the elderly [18] were used as measurement indices. They could not measure the effects of problems on the part of caregivers, such as prejudice, although they measured the extent to which disability on the part of the elderly affected dialog. Prejudices are cognitive distortions formed by nurses' internal experiences that negatively influence care and are expected to improve with education. Therefore, the following evaluation scales had been considered as indicators for the side facing the elderly.

Young people's beliefs in communication have been measured [19], but they have not addressed the influence of interlocutors' attitudes and prejudices. The use of existing social skill scales [20, 21] and communication skill scales [22, 23] was attempted in Japan. Kiss-18 is a behavioral index of social skills in dialog relationships, and communication scales developed in Japan include Nagano's [24] evaluation scale for micro-skills training and Ueno's [25] 2003 communication skills scale. Scales are available, but none of them considered the effects of aging as a problem.

The English literature presented a Kogan Scale. The Kogan Scale [26] can measure dialog attitudes influenced by prejudiced attitudes toward the elderly; hence, adopting it as the Japanese language is possible.

However, prejudiced attitudes toward the elderly consider the cognitive influence; thus, considering the kind of cultural influence the subject is receiving and causing cognitive distortion upon evaluation is necessary. Palmer points out that the Japanese view of the elderly is unique regarding the cognitive characteristics of the Japanese toward the elderly. Palmore [27] states that the Japanese government has established Respect for the Aged Day, unlike people in other countries. Concurrently, he points out that the attitude to evaluation scales proposed by other cultures cannot be applied to Japanese people who have such ambivalent attitudes toward the elderly. Therefore, the author developed a scale to measure Japanese people's dialog attitudes with the elderly, considering culturally influenced prejudiced attitudes.

## 5. Evaluation of care attitudes of nurses in geriatric nursing

### 5.1 Characteristics of evaluation scales

Shimizu developed the Dialog Preference Scales for the Elderly (DPSE or Shimizu scale), which assesses nurses' negative cognition and attitude tendencies during their conversations with elderly individuals, to help address the problem of ageism among caregivers [28].

DPSE has four subconcepts that reliably assess respondents' relationships with older people [29] (**Table 1**). These subconcepts are bewilderment (shown through uncertainty), anxiety, cognitive bias (associated with ageism), and difficulty in communication. No other standardized scale is comparable to the DPSE. However, concurrent validity was detected for the DPSE's "anxiety in relationships" item and the "authoritative anxiety" item in the Social Anxiety Scale in Social Situations [30]. Additionally, DPSE demonstrated predictive validity for the targeted achievement level for nursing students' clinical training. The total coefficient of reliability (α) was 0.811, thereby confirming internal consistency reliability. The coefficients of reliability (α) were 0.764, 0.687, 0.671, and 0.670 for bewilderment, anxiety, cognitive bias, and communication difficulty, respectively [29]. This scale requires careful interpretation of the scores because the total score represents the degree of negative aspects of attitudes.

### 5.2 Characteristics of nurses' interactive attitudes with the elderly: in comparison with nursing students

We clarified the characteristics of nurses' interactive attitudes with the elderly in comparison with nursing students. This is a finding obtained from a survey of Japanese nurses and nursing students.

Data collection was conducted at hospitals and seminars in Japan. Participants were nurses (n = 186; males: 2.7%; females: 97.3%) and nursing students [n = 552; males: 2.0% (38.4 ± 10.3 years); females: 98.0% (22.9 ± 4.9 years)]. Nursing student data from a study with the same questionnaire were obtained retrospectively.

Data were gathered using the 15-item Shimizu Scale, which measures attributes and four subconcepts (bewilderment, anxiety, cognitive bias, and communication difficulty). Higher scores indicate more negative cognitions or attitudes (maximum score: 28). Data were descriptively analyzed using t-tests and secondary factor analysis of confirmatory factors. The responses of nurses were compared with the previously collected responses of nursing students who differed from nurses in their experience and knowledge.

Nurses' total scores (mean: 3.94) were significantly lower than the nursing students' scores (mean: 4.4), indicating that nurses had a more positive view of communication with older people than nursing students.

The path coefficients for dialog preferences in the subfactor for nurses were 0.48 for bewilderment, 0.36 for anxiety, 0.34 for cognitive bias, and 0.72 for communication difficulty (**Figure 1**). When comparing the fit of the subconcept analysis model,

| | | |
|---|---|---|
| 1. Sex () | | |
| 2. Age () | | |
| 3. Clinical experience (years) () | | |
| 4. Have you experienced living with older people? (Presently yes/In the past yes/no) | | |
| Please respond to the questions using the following scale that assumes that the distance between numbers is equal. Circle one number (1–7) that best represents your opinion: 1 (Strongly disagree)—2—3—4 (Neither agree nor disagree) —5—6—7 (Strongly agree). | | |
| No | Questions | Grading (6-point Likert type) 1: strongly disagree, 7: strongly agree |
| 1 | I am aware of a major age gap with older clients and find it difficult to think of suitable topics of conversation. | 1—2—3—4—5—6—7 |
| 2 | I am uncertain how seriously I should listen to older clients. | 1—2—3—4—5—6—7 |
| 3 | I always try to maintain a loud voice when I talk to older clients, so I tend to say things that are not really what I want to say. | 1—2—3—4—5—6—7 |
| 4 | I do not know how to react when older clients repeat themselves. | 1—2—3—4—5—6—7 |
| 5 | In conversation, when older clients talk about history, I am not sure what to do because my knowledge is limited. | 1—2—3—4—5—6—7 |
| 6 | I worry about the vision of older clients. How do they see and how much do they see? | 1—2—3—4—5—6—7 |
| 7 | When talking to older clients, I wonder whether my voice is the right volume and if my tone is appropriate. | 1—2—3—4—5—6—7 |
| 8 | When talking to older clients, I worry that I may exhaust them. | 1—2—3—4—5—6—7 |
| 9 | I wonder how older clients view us, the young generation. | 1—2—3—4—5—6—7 |
| 10 | Older clients just want someone to listen to them all the time. | 1—2—3—4—5—6—7 |
| 11 | Older clients want somebody to listen to them and they want to talk about themselves. | 1—2—3—4—5—6—7 |
| 12 | It seems that once older clients start talking they often do not stop. | 1—2—3—4—5—6—7 |
| 13 | It is difficult to know how to speak to and deal with older clients who have dementia. | 1—2—3—4—5—6—7 |
| 14 | I find it hard to hold conversations with older clients with hearing difficulties. | 1—2—3—4—5—6—7 |
| 15 | I find it hard to communicate with older clients with total aphasia. | 1—2—3—4—5—6—7 |

**Table 1.**
*Dialog preference scales for elderly questionnaire (DPSE or Shimizu scale).*

GFI was 0.91(0.95 for nursing students), AGFI was 0.88 (0.93), and CFI was 0.94 (0.94) for nurses, indicating good model fit for nurses. However, a significant difference was seen in the apprehension score for nurses with <1-year experience compared

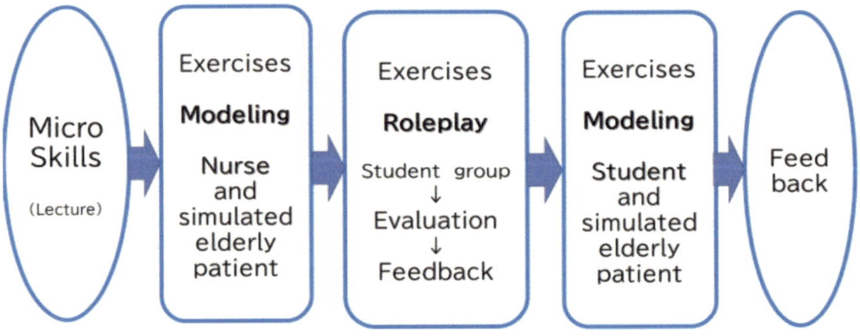


**Figure 1.**
*Training program for interactive attitudes with older people.*

with those with more experience ($p < 0.05$). Overall, compared with the nursing student data previously measured using the same scale [28], experienced nurses had more positive attitudes toward older people on the Shimizu Scale.

Moreover, a significant difference in the anxiety scores was observed between nurses with <1 year of experience and those with more experience. Experienced nurses had a more positive attitude regarding communication with older people compared with nursing students. Since this result instructed the current research results, the Shimizu Scale is appropriate for nurses.

The results of this survey show that nurses tend to have more positive attitudes toward the elderly than nursing students and first-year nurses. This is thought to be because the explanatory power of the subordinate concepts of the scale makes it possible to deal with patients with more difficult medical conditions and knowledge of the elderly, thereby reducing anxiety and preventing confusion (31).

### 5.3 Characteristics of nurses' interactive attitudes with the elderly in comparison with care workers

Nurses' interactive attitudes toward the elderly became more positive depending on their experience [31].

What is the difference between nurses and caregivers?

Nurses' and care workers' scores on the Dialog Preference Scales for Elderly (DPSE) created from data from nursing students in Japan are compared. For this forward-looking, quantitative, questionnaire-based study, data collection was conducted from 2010 to 2012 with care seminar participants in Japan.

Participants were nurses ($n = 277$; $36.96 \pm 10.33$ years old, males; 4.33% females; 95.66%) and care workers ($n = 83$; $40.52 \pm 11.68$ years old, males; 25.30% females; 74.69). The samples varied significantly in mean age ($p < 0.05$) and gender ($p < 0.001$). The number of years of experience was 139.94 for nurses with $SD = 10.99$ and 90.99 for care workers with $SD = 45.44$ ($p < 0.001$).

Data were gathered using the 15-item Dialog Preference Scales for Elderly (DPSE or Shimizu scale), which assesses nurses' negative cognition and attitude tendencies during their conversations with elderly individuals [31]. The DPSE measures attributes and the four subconcepts such as bewilderment, anxiety, cognitive bias, and communication difficulty. Higher scores indicate more negative cognitions or attitudes (maximum score: 28). Data were descriptively analyzed using Pearson's $\chi^2$ test and student's t-test of confirmatory factors.

Nurses' total scores (mean; 57.31, SD = 11.84) were not significantly different than care worker's scores (mean; 57.58, SD = 12.25), indicating that nurses and care workers had a similar view of communicating with older people. However, the subconcept of cognitive bias was significantly lower for nurses, as they likely had higher levels of ageism ($p < 0.10$).

Additionally, the communication difficulty subconcept also was significantly higher for nurses, possibly because they had been caring for much older patients with more severe illnesses ($p < 0.01$) [31].

Why do nurses have negative interactive attitudes when caring for the seriously ill elderly?

The reason is that other research results show that medical professionals have a protective attitude toward patients [32]. The protective attitude of medical staff based on the principle of health supremacy is a problem for medical staff in general. Murata et al. revealed that the possibility that nurses have this negative tendency cannot be denied. Negative views of the elderly include prejudices (Ageism) that affect words and actions [27].

## 6. An effective interactive learning method for geriatric nursing

Factors affecting the quality of nurses' care for the elderly include prejudiced dialog attitudes, in addition to negative views on the elderly, and protective attitudes. Therefore, learning is necessary to affirm this dialog attitude.

The next section will introduce the learning method.

### 6.1 Program content

The dialog training program [33] for nursing students who have completed the following pre-learning is introduced. Preparatory learning was positioned at the stage of deepening understanding of the elderly by completing the basic knowledge of basic nursing and practical training for understanding patients and receiving lectures on the elderly for 10 h.

The structure of the program consists of four elements. First, a model demonstration between an experienced nurse and a trained elderly simulated patient is viewed [33–36]. Second, students will role-play with each other. Third, a third-party evaluator and a simulated patient will evaluate the student's performance. Fourth, the performer student receives feedback from the evaluator and the simulated patient. Here, the simulated patient should verbalize and convey the patient's inner feelings. A trained simulated patient is a citizen who has the experience of being an elderly patient and who acts like a patient according to the acting scenario created under the learning objectives. Therefore, the citizen's condition is to be a learning cooperator and to express linguistically the patient-likeness of the elderly. The patient-like expression means having a sense that only the patient can be aware of and being able to verbalize it at the level of student understanding.

### 6.2 Training method

The following are the specific training methods.

The program consists of lectures and exercises. Lectures for 45 min focused on the involvement techniques of the micro-skills hierarchy constructed by Allen Ivey [37].

The exercise consists of three stages. The scenario is a geriatric scenario for a simulated geriatric patient. The first stage of the exercise is the actual model performance. A model performance of a nurse counselor and a simulated elderly patient is performed for 15 min according to the elderly scenario. At this time, the students will observe and the teacher will explain the involvement behavior and the use of micro-techniques after the implementation. The second stage involves small group role-plays of four students. Students take on the role of nurse, patient, recorder, and evaluator, and the entire group changes roles. The theme of the scenario is "Recently Worrying," and the performance is recorded for 5 min. The student receives 2 min of feedback from the evaluator after completing the performance. The evaluator gives feedback using the evaluation form for the frequency of use of the micro-techniques and the mayor's video images and recorded voices used by the recorder. This is done reciprocally. The third stage is a 15-min role-play between a student representative and a simulated patient. Students observe this and receive feedback from performers. Here, questions about the difference in feelings are asked and answered by the visiting students. Finally, the teacher summarizes the learning and concludes (**Figure 1**).

### 6.3 Effects of training

We surveyed the results of implementing an interactive learning program for the elderly with 48 nursing students [33].

After the exercise, students stated its worth because they are learning (100%), they understood the actual atmosphere, attitudes, and postures (29%), and they learned more about non-verbal communication, communication selection, and interaction. Of the respondents, 29% understood the content of the lecture through role-playing and feedback, 29% understood the content of the lecture, and 19% thought of it as a useful learning experience as it reduced their anxiety. As for the simulated patients, 95% stated a good practice experience of participating in the simulated patients. This is supported by the following statements: "the model performance gave me an atmosphere that I could not capture with videotapes or lectures," "I experienced different viewpoints through role-playing," and "feedback from a tape recorder made my reflections more effective." Additionally, "I was surprised by the simulated patient's appearance," "I could not clarify the difference between paraphrasing and closed questions," "I felt a real tension in the nurse counselor's skillful technique, Speaking," "I was able to see the depth of my habits," "I was able to see my habits objectively," and "Students' feedback helped me understand." These descriptions suggest that the program was effective.

The statistical examination revealed that the items before and after program learning were significantly "clarified clues for non-verbal communication." This is supported by the following statements: "the other person's intentions are reflected in the non-verbal communication that naturally occurs in the process of empathizing with them," "the silence that affects the first meeting and the first impression has meaning," "the anxiety of communication is reduced," etc. Therefore, through this type of learning, students will reduce their anxiety about interacting with the elderly and reduce their expressions of embarrassment.

## 7. Conclusion

Japan has the highest rate of the aging population in the OECD. Moreover, Japan has rapidly become an aging society in a short period compared to countries such as

France. In Asia, South Korea and Singapore are also aging faster than Japan. In 2000, Japan developed a Long-Term Care Insurance Law for the financial security of elderly care, called the Long-term Care Insurance Law. Twenty-two years have passed since its inception, and it continues to utilize the Long-Term Care Insurance Act with some modifications. Japan's elderly care methods, including the Nursing Care Insurance Law, will serve as a reference for countries that will become aging societies in the future.

In this chapter, it was explained that young caregivers requires to understand as old people who lived in an unknown past, to understand the physical and psychological changes that accompany aging, and to understand the attitudes of caregivers themselves. As a way of solving problems, the attitudes of nurses were evaluated, and improving the quality of care with undistorted attitudes was explained, as well as specific teaching methods.

I recommend that caregivers, in a country that is becoming an aging society, use this as a reference and hope that they will contribute to the successful aging of the elderly.

## Acknowledgements

The Dialog Preference Scales for Elderly Questionnaire developed and described by the author in this chapter is the author's doctoral dissertation. Japan is notorious for its aging society, but there is no bachelor's degree in gerontology in Japan. However, due to the need for gerontological research, J. F. Oberlin University, a private school, established a gerontology major in its graduate school of international studies. The author's doctorate in gerontology was registered as one of the first gerontologists in Japan. Professors Masami Nojiri of the Honorary professor of Chiba University, Professor Hisao Osada and Professor Hidehiro Sugisawa of Oberin University, and Professor Masahiro Kodama of the University of Tsukuba supervised this doctoral dissertation. I would like to express my gratitude to my mentor.

This study was supported by Enago and the Program to supporting research activities of female researchers by MEXT (Ministry of Education, Culture, Sports, Science and Technology) in in manuscript submission.

## Conflict of interest

The authors declare no conflict of interest.

## Author details

R.N. Hiroko Shimizu
Faculty of Medicine, Kagawa University, Kita-Gun, Kagawa, Japan

*Address all correspondence to: shimizu.hiroko@kagawa-u.ac.jp

## References

[1] Rowe JW, Kahn RL. Human aging: Usual and successful. Science. 1987;**37**:143-149

[2] Karasawa A. Mental functioning of older people. In: Tomonaga M, Sato A, editors. Aging of the Brain and Nervous System. Tokyo: Asakura Shoten; 1989

[3] Butler RN. Age-ism: Another form of bigotry. Gerontologist. 1969;**9**:243-246

[4] Butler RN. Ageism. In: Maddox GL, editor. The Encyclopaedia of Aging, New York. NY: Springer; 1995

[5] Palmore EB. Types of ageism. In: Palmore EB, editor. Ageism: Negative and Positive. New York, NY: Springer Publishing Company, Inc; 1999

[6] Baba J. Old man view of junior high school students-Measurement using old man view scale. Social Gerontology. 1993;**38**:3-12

[7] Statistics Bureau, Ministry of Internal Affairs and Communications of Japan. Population estimates. 2021. Available from: https://www.stat.go.jp/data/jinsui/2021np/index.html [Accessed:2022-Oct. 29]

[8] Ministry of Health, Labor and Welfare of Japan. Overview of vital statistics (confirmed numbers) of Japanese. 2021. Available from: https://www.mhlw.go.jp/toukei/saikin/hw/jinkou/kakutei21/dl/15_all.pdf [Accessed:2022-Oct. 29]

[9] Ministry of Economy. Trade and Industry, OECD (Organization for Economic Co-operation and Development). 2022. Available from: https://www.meti.go.jp/policy/trade_policy/oecd/index.html [Accessed:2022-Oct. 29]

[10] OECD. Elderly population. 2022. Available from: https://data.oecd.org/pop/elderly-population.html [Accessed: 2022-Oct. 29]

[11] Cabinet Office of Japan. White Paper on the Aging Society (whole version). 2020

[12] Foundation for Promotion of Longevity Science of Japan. Healthy Longevity Net. 2022. Available from: https://www.tyojyu.or.jp/net/byouki/frailty/about.html [Accessed:2022-Oct. 29]

[13] Cabinet Office of Japan. White Paper on the Aging Society, (whole version 2) International Trends in Aging. 2020. Available from: https://www8.cao.go.jp/kourei/whitepaper/w-2020/html/zenbun/s1_1_2.html [Accessed:2022-Oct. 29]

[14] The Institute of Tokyo Metropolitan Geriatrics and Gerontology. Homepage of the Institute of Tokyo Metropolitan Geriatrics and Gerontology. 2020. Available from: https://www.tmghig.jp/research/release/2020/0903.html [Accessed:2022-Oct. 29]

[15] Foundation for Promotion of Longevity Science. Healthy Longevity Net. 2022. Available from: https://www.tyojyu.or.jp/net/index.html [Accessed:2022-Oct. 29]

[16] Shiotsuka W, Burton GU, Pedretti LW, et al. An examination of performance scores on activities of daily living between elders with right and left cerebrovascular accident. Physical & Occupational Therapy in Geriatrics. 1992;**10**(4):47-57

[17] Rankin EJ. Bed side evaluation of learning and memory: Descriptive information on a shortened version of

the Luria memory words test. Journal of Clinical Psychology. 2000;**56**:113-118

[18] Erber NP, Holland J, Osborn RR. Communicating with elders: Effects of speaker-listener distance. British Journal of Audiology. 1998;**32**:135-138

[19] McCann RM, Cargile AC, Giles H, et al. Communication ambivalence toward elders: Data from North Vietnam, South Vietnam, and the U.S.A. Journal of Cross-Cultural Gerontology. 2004;**19**:275-297

[20] Hondo K. Using her SST to improve communication skills of nurses. Transactions of the Japanese Society of Nursing (Nursing Management). 2007;**37**:409-411

[21] Kusaka T, Soya T, Ageno Y. Nursing students' interpersonal relationship Research on psychiatric nursing skills after completion of clinical training in psychiatric nursing, Prosecutor. Bulletin of Kawasaki College of Medical Sciences. 2005;**25**:29-34

[22] Kido T, Shiomi M, Takami K, et al. Evaluating the communication skills of her nursing students using the communication skills scale (NCSI), her NCS comparison and evaluation factors in her 3rd year and her 2nd year. Bulletin of Nursing School Attached to Osaka Medical College. 2005;**11**:8-12

[23] Kido T, Takami K, Shiomi M. Evaluation of nursing students' communication ability using the communication skills scale (NCSI) Comparison of 2nd and 3rd year students at 7 schools. Bulletin of Nursing School Attached to Osaka Medical College. 2004;**10**:1-5

[24] Nagano H, Hasegawa M, Tori F, et al. A study on the preparation of the empathic understanding scale EUS self-evaluation table. An attempt to improve selling techniques, Shizuoka Prefectural Nursing College Special Research Report 2013-2014. 2003. pp. 1-25

[25] Ueno R. Analysis of communication skill evaluation items (No. 2) Examination of reliability and validity. Akien Prefecture Nursing Education Research Society Journal. 2003;**28**:27-33

[26] Kogan N. Attitudes toward old people: The development of a scale and an examination of correlates. Journal of Abnormal and Social Psychology. 1961;**62**:44-54

[27] Palmore EB. translated by Suzuki K. 2002. Ageism: The Reality of Age Discrimination and Prospects for Overcoming It. Tokyo: Akashi Shoten; 1999. pp. 43-84

[28] Shimizu H. The problems and characteristics of communication between nursing students and the elderly. Journal of Japan Academy of Gerontological Nursing. 2007;**11**:56-63

[29] Shimizu H. Validity and reliability of dialogue preference scales for elders. Journal of Japan Academy of Gerontological Nursing. 2010;**14**:34-41

[30] Mori I, Tanno Y. Reliability and validity of creating social anxiety scale in social situations scale. Journal of Health Research. 2001;**14**:23-31

[31] Shimizu H. Comparison of Japanese nurses' and care workers' scores on the dialogue preference scales for elderly (DPSE). International Journal of Nursing & Clinical Practices. 2021;**7**:328

[32] Gekoski W, Knex V. Ageism or Healthism?: Perceptions Based on Age and Health Status. Journal of Ageing Health. Journal of Aging Health. 1990;**2**:15-27

[33] Shimizu H, Nojiri M. Characteristics of an educational program for elderly communication for students using simulated patients. Human Care Research. 2005;**6**:45-54

[34] Shimizu H, Yokoi I, Toyoda S, et al. Characteristics of studies on simulated patients and standardized patients in nursing education. Journal of the Japanese Society of Health Sciences. 2008;**10**:215-223

[35] Shimizu H. Utilization of simulated patients in nursing education characteristics and evaluation of simulated patients. Perspectives on Nursing. 2009a;**34**:68-70

[36] Shimizu H. Utilization of simulated patients in nursing education ingenuity and implementation method of utilizing simulated patients in nursing - objective-based participatory learning of simulated patients. Nursing Perspectives. 2009b;**34**:69-72

[37] Ivey AE translated Fukuhara M, Kajiyama K, Kokubu H, Nireki M. Introduction to Microcounseling. USA: Cole Publishing Company, A Division of Wadsworth Inc; 1985. p. 8

Chapter 2

# Reflective Approaches in Nursing Education and Clinical Practice

*Geeta Parwanda*


## Abstract

Today modern society is becoming more complex and constantly information is changing along with problem solving strategies, reflective learning is an ability to look **back** over an **experience** and break it down into its significant aspects, such as any factors affecting success or failure. Due to this complex and continually changing environment, healthcare professionals could benefit from a program of reflective practice. Reflective Practice (DAVIS 2012) 1 is increasing from an experience for any situation, acquisition of new knowledge and skills, further understanding of own beliefs, attitudes and values. This practice involves encouragement of self-motivation and self-directed learning in nursing education and clinical practice.


**Keywords:** reflective practice, nursing education, clinical practice, health care professional, reflective approaches

## 1. Introduction

Today Modern society is becoming more complex since the Covid-19 pandemic starts the information is becoming more advanced with technology and changing more rapidly leading users to constantly rethink, moving to new direction and adopt problem solving strategies.

Reflective learning is a capacity to **look back** over an **experience** and able to analysis in significant way, any factors which affect success or failure.

Learning in reflection will aid in enhancement for own human skill development and finding a clear path between the effort in development activity and outcome of it Reflection also heap in knowing are learning experiences regarding the purpose of activity and its importance (**Figure 1**). Reflecting on learning enables to link professional development to practical outcomes and widens the definition of what counts as useful activity.

Being is learner in reflective practice. One always try to apply knowledge and practice in further work as learning is always connected to the action and theoretical knowledge to clinical skills.

We can always assess our learning outcome through the feedback from peer group teachers with self assessment. As we understated that reflection is the process which aid to gain meaningful look into are professional practice.

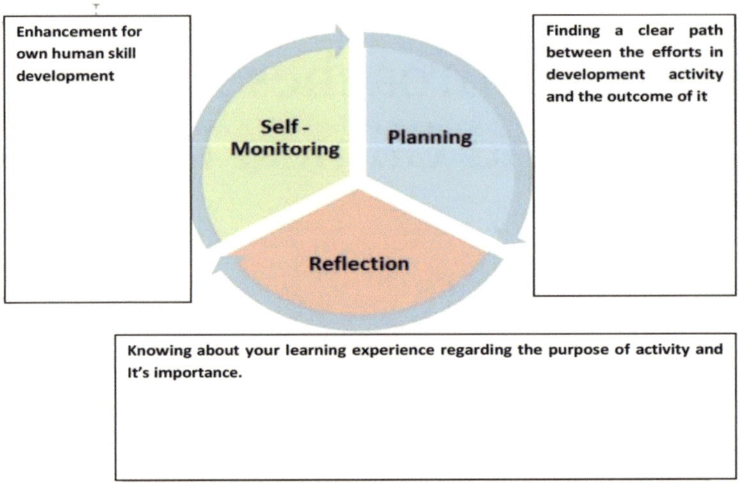


**Figure 1.**
*Learning in reflection.*

## 2. Reflective approaches

In nursing education reflective approaches can be used as important tool in clinical practice based where the nursing student learn from their own professional experience, classrooms lecture or mentor which is always helpful in career advancement and adopting same process is able to bring together theory and clinical practice.

As Paterson Chapman [1, 2] mentioned that reflection is vital part of learning from experience and mainly lead to develop and maintain completely across a professional's lifetime in the area of health care. John Dewey was among the first to explain about Reflective Practice with his exploration of experience, connection between incidents as shown in **Figure 2**.

Reflections helps to see and able to mark schools of thought and theory of concept within the context of our work done [3]. Important point to be noted about reflection during the practice reveals that the individual not only look back on his past activities and the action taken, but also deeply look into observation of emotions shown, previous happenings, actions taken, and its effect and thus lead to higher level of understanding [2].

The use of reflection in nursing education:

1. Enhance self awareness leader to increases understanding of the effect that past experience may have on care delivery.

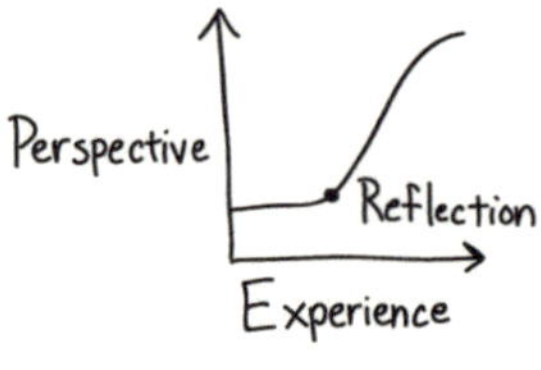


**Figure 2.**
*Experience and reflective process.*

2. To develop nursing students intellectual capacities to conceptualize knowledge to better assess client need.

3. Acquiring of novice knowledge and clinical practice skill.

4. Analysis of self and value, core, belief and attitude.

### 2.1 The various model of reflective practice

Reflective practice applied in disciplines such as teaching, nursing, social work as a way to learn from real life experience. There are many models to explain and guide personal and situational analysis and improvement. The first stage of reflection usually start with the description what has happened and the next stage of reflective practice describe about what we know the situation and what it is impact and the final stage of reflection briefs about the change and outcome of situation as explained in **Figure 3** the co-relation of Reflection, learning and action. The structure and format of these modals may have difference but mostly all reflective modals have many common features.

#### *2.1.1 Gibbs' reflective cycle or Gibbs' model of reflection (1988)*

One of the most common cyclical models of reflection which consist of following six distinct stages of exploring the experience [4].

- Description
- Feelings
- Evaluation
- Analysis
- Conclusions
- Action plan.

Gibbs reflective cycle allows to reflect upon ones experience as they happen and it helps to enhance our performance and for better improvement in future.

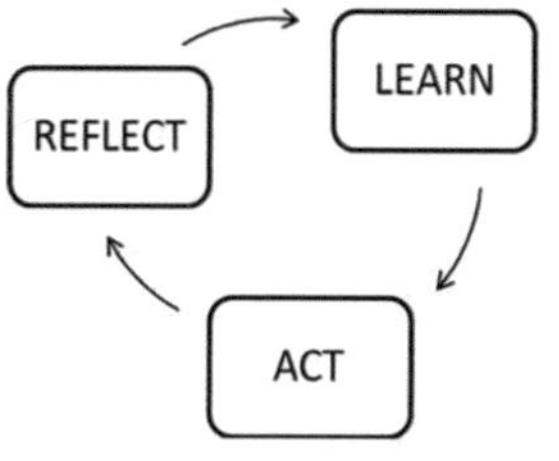


**Figure 3.**
*Co-relation of reflection, learning and action.*

*2.1.2 Rolfe 2001*

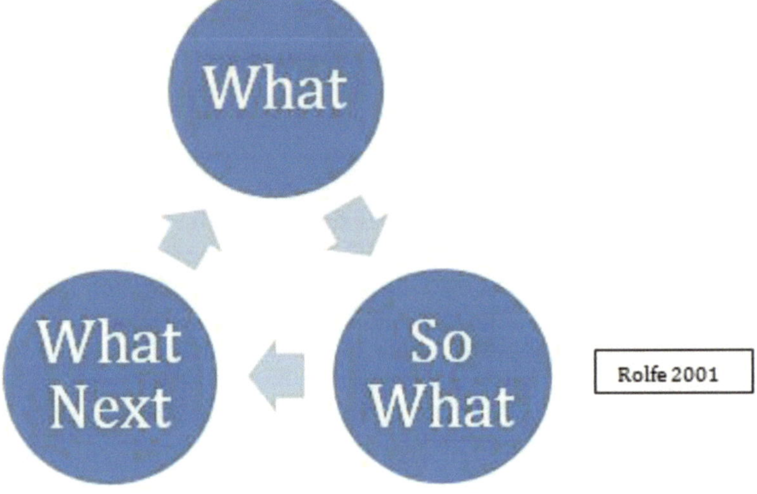


**Figure 4.**
*Rolfe reflective framework.*

## 2.2 Adaptation of the Rolfe reflective model

Rolfe's reflective model is based on three simple questions what happened, (self awareness) and how it happened (critical analysis and evaluation), and what will be next plan (action oriented), so what and what next (As shown in **Figure 4**). A simplistic cycle composed of three questions which asks the practitioner, by introducing the problem that they are reflecting on before making their observation about the issue and finally concluding what they would change next time Through this analysis, a description of the situation is given which leads into the scrutiny of the situation and the construction of knowledge that has been learn through the experience. The most important advantage of Rolfe model relates to its clarity and simplicity. It often produce meaningful solutions.This models not only consider reflection after the moment but when the event is taking place so that the corrective measure can be taken.

To conclude Rolfe model describe that reflections does not remain superficial but it is comprehensive by completing the simple action plan with key pointers about what we will do and how will decide that our practice has improved.

*2.2.1 Ganshirt 2007*

The reflective model Christian Ganshirt 2007 was prepared on the concept of the design cycle and the Ganshirt design cycle is explained with the first step begin with any innovative thoughts and next step is using visual and audio aids through same ideas is expressed and transfer in cyclical way with the critical rethinking and the same process goes on.

To summarize these models provide a useful guide or mode to begin but reflection is a unique and innate process and nursing professional will perceive it in a different way. Everyone takes some time to try different reflective approaches until it works positive and effective.As the time passes and as a reflective practitioner that we may try to practice different methods to handle the current situation.

The main four level of reflection can be described as:-

1. Response to any situation.

2. Exploration of learner response to same situation.

3. Analysis of the response and by investigating the action taken.

4. Indentify the outcome for the future clinical practice.

### 2.3 Application of reflective learning for health professional

Reflective Practice is always connected with learning from previous experience, and is considered as an important strategy for nursing professionals who believes in learning process in all phases of lives and it is known fact there is always changes in context of healthcare practices leading to continuous progression in medical knowledge hence there is a always remarkable need for experts in medical and nursing education.

Reflective practices seem to be important tool for healthcare professional because of rapid changes in healthcare facilities. Price explained in 2004 [5] about the benefits of reflective practices for healthcare practitioner by understanding his or her own motive,thoughts,moral and feelings connected with client care and to promote solution to practice situations and meet challenge with existing ideas, response of action taken with positive or negative feeling and also to rethink how the practice situation can be handled in different way.

In the field of nursing profession there is always a concern that actions taken in any situation may have the risk of habitualization, thus dehumanizing client care and their needs. Reflective Practice always aids to nurses are to plan their process of nursing care and keen monitoring the action to ensure it is beneficial to the clients.

The act of reflection is seen as a way of promoting the self decision, qualified and professionals with leadership quality. Involving in Reflective Practice leads to the improvement of the quality of nursing care, enhancing personal and professional growth and reducing the gap between theory and practice. Reflective practices are now being introduced into undergraduate, postgraduate and continuing nursing education. Mann [6] expressed in her research that in nursing professional in clinical practice reflection process is multi factorial and to include different aspects. All experiences during anticipation of a difficult situation also added to reflection. Practicing professionals always have variation in their attitudes and capability to reflect. Denner [7] mentioned that reflection has meditation aspect which causes a change in brain alpha and theta wave activity and also increases the right hemisphere brain activity which is connected to our insights and leads to sudden awareness of correct answer to any verbal problem and leads to creativity. Many researchers have proved that self reflection involves the brain's cortical midline structures (CMS) any disturbance to the CMS causes difficulty in evaluating the difficult situation and there is tendency to overestimate one's personal abilities [8].

## 3. Conclusion

To prevent burnout, nursing professional need to have passion of their profession. Nursing professional at every level after this covid 19 pandemic will need to be more perseverant and passionate with excellence in clinical practice [9]. Thus reflective learning is important tool to learn and enhance skill competency over time and evaluates our learning experience towards nursing care. Self reflection enhances skills which involve motivation and temperament which are necessary for success in the health care professional.

## Acknowledgements

I would like to acknowledge the extraordinary debt I owe to the editor and my special thanks to Paula Gavran, Author Service manager for her continual support. I also thanks to all my reader.

## Conflict of interest

I declare no conflict of interest.

## Further reading

- Dewey J. How We Think. Revised ed. Boston: D.C Heath; 1933
- Schön D. The Reflective Practitioner, How Professionals Think in Action. Basic Books; 1983
- Hartman HJ. Teaching Metacognitively. In: Metacognition in Learning and Instruction. Dordrecht: Springer; 2001
- Freshwater D, Horton-Deutsch S, Sherwood G, Taylor B. Resource Paper: The Scholarship of Reflective Practice. The Honor Society of Nursing, Sigma Theta Tau International; 2005

## Author details

Geeta Parwanda
Faculty of Nursing, Swami Vivekananda Subharti University, Meerut, Uttarpardesh, India

*Address all correspondence to: parwandaa@yahoo.com

## References

[1] Samantha D. Embracing reflective practice. Education for Primary Care. 2012;**23**(1):9-12

[2] Chapman P. Enhancing skills of critical reflection to evidence learning in professional practice. National Library of Medicine. 2013;**13**(3):133-138

[3] McBrien B. Learning from practice-reflections on a critical incident. Accident and Emergency Nursing. 2007;**15**(3):128-133. DOI: 10.1016/j.aaen.2007.03.004 Epub 2007 May 30

[4] Gibbs G. Learning by doing: A guide to teaching and learning methods. London: Oxford Centre for Staff and Learning Development, Oxford Polytechnic, Further Education Unit; 1988

[5] Price A. Encouraging reflection and critical thinking in practice. Nursing Standard. 2004;**18**(47):46-52, quiz 53-4. DOI: 10.7748/ns2004.08.18.47.46.c3664

[6] Mann K. Reflection and reflective practice in health profession education. Advances in Health Sciences Education Theory Practice. 2009;**14**(4):595-621

[7] Denner SS. The science of energy therapies and contemplative practice. A conceptual review and application of zero balancing. Holistic Nursing Practice. 2009;**23**(6):315-334

[8] Van der Meer L, Costafreda S, Aleman A, David AS. Self-reflection and the brain: A theoretical review and meta-analysis of neuroimaging studies with implications for schizophrenia. Neuroscience and Biobehavioral Reviews. 2010;**34**(6):936-946

[9] Turale S et al. Challenging times: Ethics, nursing and the COVID-19 pandemic. International Nursing Review. 2020;**67**(2):164-167. DOI: 10.1111/inr.12598

**Chapter 3**

# Starting Somewhere: Advanced Practice Nursing in Canada

*Sarah A. Balcom*


## Abstract

Many countries are capitalizing on nurses with advanced degrees or practice experience to increase patients' access to healthcare. In Canada, there are two advanced practice nursing roles – nurse practitioners (NPs) and clinical nurse specialists (CNS). While both NPs and CNSs are knowledgeable nursing leaders who make important contributions to the healthcare system, only NPs have a protected title and are separately licensed from registered nurses (RNs). In this chapter, the author explores how entry-level-competencies (ELCs) are essential to the separate licensure of NPs. The author also argues how ELCs may increase NPs' role recognition and effective use in the Canadian healthcare system.


**Keywords:** nurse practitioners, clinical nurse specialists, registered nurses, nursing education, teaching and assessment

## 1. Introduction

"If you don't start somewhere, you're going to go nowhere." – Bob Marley.

Globally, registered nurses (RNs) with advanced degrees or specialized qualifications often take on important clinical leadership and advanced practice roles, which can increase patients' access to quality healthcare [1]. However, the context and implementation of these roles varies between countries, with some countries showing slower acceptance and/or implementation than others [1, 2]. In one study, Jean et al. [2] explored advanced nursing roles in Canada and Spain, and found that, while both countries needed these roles, each country was at a different implementation stage. Similar barriers to implementation were found in both countries, including lack of role clarity, opposition from other health professionals (e.g., concerns about 'scope creep' or the scope of practice expansion of one health profession through legislation into the scope of practice of another), education/training issues, and regulatory concerns [2]. These findings are similar to those of other researchers [3, 4].

Entry-level competencies (ELCs), written collaboratively by advanced practice nurses, regulatory bodies and other stakeholders, including other health professionals and patients, increase the role clarity and integration of one advanced practice nursing role, that of the nurse practitioner (NP), into the healthcare system [5]. These statements describe the abilities/knowledge/judgment entry-level practitioners need to provide safe care [6, 7]. ELCs provide the 'somewhere' to start for other advanced practice nurses seeking to better define and promote their roles and receive greater recognition for their contributions to quality patient care.

## 2. Canada's advanced practice nursing and nurse practitioners

The ICN [1] uses the term 'advanced practice nurse' to describe "a generalist or specialist nurse who has acquired, through additional graduate education (minimum of a master's degree), the expert knowledge base, complex decision-making skills and clinical competencies" for an expanded role in patient care (p. 6). In Canada, advanced practice nursing began in the 1890s with outpost nurses who worked in isolated, rural, and northern areas [8]. Over the years, Canadian advanced practice nursing has evolved, and today, there are two widely recognized advanced practice nursing roles – NPs and clinical nurse specialists (CNS) [9]. While NPs and CNSs are both knowledgeable nursing leaders who contribute significantly to patients' care, only NPs have a protected title and are separately licensed from RNs [10]. The first NPs in Canada appeared in the 1960s and were viewed as a solution to physician shortages, and a way to increase patients' access to primary healthcare and lower costs [11]. By 1972, a national report (the Boudreau report) recommended the implementation of NPs to meet Canadian primary healthcare needs [8]. The recommendations were not followed, and the Canada-wide implementation of NPs has remained inconsistent [12, 13].

There is strong evidence supporting NPs' effectiveness as care providers in a variety of settings. Stanik-Hutt et al. [14] reviewed 37 articles published between 1990 and 2009 and determined that NP-provided care was on par with physician-provided care in primary care clinics. Kleinpell et al. [15] reviewed 53 articles between 2008 and 2018 and concluded that the evidence supported the inclusion of NPs in the care of acute and even critically ill patients. Despite the number of studies illustrating the value of NPs as care providers, the implementation of the role Canada-wide has been variable [13]. The role is most widely implemented in Ontario [16]. In 2021, there were 7400 active NP licenses in Canada, with over half practicing in Ontario [16].

## 3. Barriers to implementation

Several studies have identified barriers or factors that impede the implantation of the NP role across Canada [17–21]. The most common barrier noted in these studies relates to role clarity. For example, Kilpatrick et al. [18], who evaluated the integration of NPs into a cardiology healthcare team in Quebec, found NPs struggled to practice to their full scope due to unclear role definition. They noted that this may also have contributed to tension between NPs and other team members, particularly physicians [18]. As Rickards and Hamilton [19] note, a lack of role clarity can lead to confusion among patients and other team members, hindering collaboration and effective implementation of the role. Role confusion is understandable. In Canada, NPs' roles are determined by both their legal and individual scopes of practice. The legal NP scope of practice (i.e., what NPs are authorized to do) is defined through provincial legislation (i.e., nursing acts), with NP roles expanding in many provinces over the years [9]. In Ontario, for example, NP's authority to prescribe prior to 2010 was restricted to a pre-approved list of drugs or renewing drugs first prescribed by physicians [22]. Since then, their prescribing privileges have expanded to more classes of drugs, including controlled drugs/substances [22]. Today, all provinces and territories have NP legislation in place [9]. Although there is some variation, generally, NPs can autonomously diagnose/treat diseases, order/interpret tests, prescribe medications, and perform procedures [9].

Individual NPs' scopes of practice may differ from their legal scopes of practice; and may be influenced by many factors, particularly their clinical competence [23]. For example, Medical Assistance in Dying (MAiD) was legalized in Canada in 2016 [24]. In most provinces, NPs are authorized to prescribe substances that cause death for eligible patients [25]. In these provinces, however, each NP must determine their clinical competency to participate in MAiD [24]. If an NP does not feel competent to participate, they may develop this through additional education/clinical experience. The concept of clinical competence is difficult to define [26]. Benner [27] defines clinical competence as the ability to perform a task to a desirable outcome under certain circumstances within a clinical context. Other authors argue that this concept needs to be considered more holistically [28, 29]. For example, Nabizadeh-Gharghozar et al. [28] explain clinical competence as "the combination of knowledge, skills, attitude and ability" which are used to provide safe patient care without supervision (p. 2). NPs' competence can be visualized as a balloon that expands and changes shape throughout their careers as they gain clinical experience and the context of their practice changes [5].

## 4. Enablers to implementation

Some studies have identified enablers or factors that facilitate the implementation of the NP role. Unsurprisingly, a scoping review by Torrens et al. [21], found that role clarity and a positive attitude by other healthcare professionals toward the clinical competency of NPs promote role implementation. Similarly, Brault et al. [30] found it was essential to clarify roles when NPs joined primary care teams to mitigate power struggles, facilitate integration, and foster intra/interprofessional collaboration.

One effort by NP-advocates and supporters to clarify the NP role was the development of ELCs for NPs. In 2012, the Canadian Council of Registered Nurse Regulators (CCRNR) began a project to establish national ELCs to standardize NP practice and improve NP mobility [6]. The resulting ELCs were organized into four categories: (1) patient care, (2) quality improvement and research, 3) leadership, and 4) education, and were adopted, with some adaptions, by nearly all provincial/territorial regulatory bodies [31]. Each of the categories is supported by specifically written statements, which describe the minimum expected levels of performance required for newly graduated NPs to practice safely in a variety of settings [7, 31]. The ELCs articulate, using standardized language, NPs' role and how their practice differs from that of other nursing professionals, such as RNs [6]. Notably, the ELCs are not static and are revised/modified to respond to current issues, needs, and trends in NP practice, such as increasing concerns about mental health and problematic substance use [31] or the recommendations from the Truth and Reconciliation Commission of Canada [32].

The ELCs increase the standardization of NP education, which is also essential for role clarity and development [33]. As Bryant Lukosius et al. [33] argue, the standardization of NP education is needed to achieve consistency and ensure curriculums align with current and expanding NP scopes of practice. In countries like Canada, where generalized nursing education is at the baccalaureate level, NPs currently require a masters degree from an accredited program. This was not always the case, as a 2010 environmental scan by the Canadian Association of Schools of Nursing [34] found that only 75% of the 27 NP programs in Canada were at the masters level. The ELCs are both a guide for curriculum development and a way for accrediting and regulatory bodies to assess NP education programs [35]. Increased standardization means that NP educators must prove to accreditors/regulators how they prepare their students to meet the ELCs [36]. Consequently, many NP educators use curriculum mapping to provide evidence that their curriculum/courses demonstrate alignment. The ELCs also inform the development and revision of the Canadian Nurse Practitioner Examination [35]. Thus, they are an essential link between formal educational programs (like master's programs) and licensing bodies (i.e., the provincial/territorial nursing regulatory bodies).

The ELCs guide both curriculum development in NP programs and entry-level exam test plans and so are critical to the NP licensure process [35]. Provincial/territorial legislation allows nursing regulatory bodies to protect the public by setting NP licensure requirements and ensuring all NPs practice at an acceptable level [37]. The NP licensure process is similar in most provinces and territories, and involves an assessment of applicants' experience, education, and competence [38]. Specifically, applicants need to prove they (1) were previously registered as an RN, (2) completed an NP educational program, and (3) passed the Canadian Nurse Practitioners Examination [38]. Licensing assures patients that they are treated by qualified professionals who will provide a safe standard of care.

## 5. Clinical nurse specialists

NPs are often confused with CNSs, the other widely recognized advanced practice nursing role [10]. Although there are similarities between the two, such as requiring advanced degrees and/or qualifications, there are important differences [33]. As Bryant-Lukosius et al. [33] emphasizes, NPs usually provide more direct patient care, while CNSs support excellence in clinical practice. The CNS title is not protected. Also, only NPs must meet ELCs specific to their role and are licensed separately from RNs [10]. Arguably, the implementation of CNSs in Canada has been even more inconsistent than NPs [10]. As Bryan-Lukosius et al. [33] notes, "the profile and deployment of CNS roles... have fluctuated ... and the full benefit of the role has yet to be realized" (p. 140). Several studies reported role confusion and role overlap with NPs as barriers [39]. Some CNS-advocates argue that ELCs specific to the CNS role may help with its advancement and the standardization of CNS education [8, 40]. However, opponents argue that ELCs are unnecessary because CNSs do not write a different licensing examination and have separate licenses from RNs [40]. These opponents also worry ELCs may not capture the multifaceted aspects of this role, which is perceived as more varied than the NP role, with more involvement supporting other healthcare providers and leading evidence-based practice, quality assurance and program development activities [40, 41].

In 2014, CNA published the "Pan-Canadian Core Competencies for the Clinical Nurse Specialist" to clarify the role. In the future, there may be separate ELCs, which describe the minimum expected levels of performance required for all CNSs new in their roles. ELCs may be 'somewhere' to start for those looking to further standardize CNS education (e.g., a specialized masters degree or certificate/diploma program), develop CNS certification exams (similar to those in the United States), or set up other special credentialing [40]. If CNS-advocates advance the role in any of these directions, ELCs will be a needed starting point.

## 6. Directions for the future

The CCRNR [35] is updating the national NP ELCs, which will guide the development of a new entry-to-practice exam. This will further increase the standardization and quality of Canadian NP educational programs. The COVID-19 pandemic showed the multiple vulnerabilities of the healthcare system and the vital role NPs can play [42]. The number of NPs grew by 10.7% between 2020 and 2021 [16]. Although the future looks bright, a shortage of qualified nurse academics may limit future student enrollments [43]. Canada, like many countries, is plagued by a recurrent nursing faculty shortage [34]. As CASN [34] report found, Canadian nursing schools could not fill 46 faculty positions, representing a 2% vacancy rate. To fully implement the NP role, qualified nursing academics are needed to educate the next generation. Future research is needed to address the factors contributing to the nursing academic workforce shortage and to develop innovative strategies to promote faculty recruitment and retention [43].

## 7. Conclusion

In Canada, implementation of the NP role has yet to be fully realized, primarily due to role confusion. This confusion has led to less awareness about the role, which has made healthcare regulators slow to take advantage of these skilled professionals. The establishment of national ELCs provides a means to articulate the role of newly graduated NPs and to ensure acceptance of their role by other health professionals and the patient community. The ELCs increase the standardization/quality of NP educational programs, guide curriculum development, are a way for accrediting and regulatory bodies to assess NP education programs and inform the development and revision of the entry-to-practice exam. Consequently, they are an essential link between formal educational programs (like masters programs) and licensing bodies (i.e., the provincial/territorial nursing regulatory bodies). CNS-advocates who want to advance the role through more standardized education or other special credentialing may want to develop similar ELCs as 'somewhere' to start.

## Author details

Sarah A. Balcom
University of New Brunswick, Canada

*Address all correspondence to: o295d@unb.ca

## References

[1] International Council of Nurses. Guidelines on advanced practice nursing: 2020. 2020. Available from: https://www.icn.ch/system/files/documents/2020-04/ICN_APN%20Report_EN_WEB.pdf

[2] Jean E, Guerra S, Contandriopoulos D, Perroux M, Kilpatrick K, Zabalegui A. Context and implementation of advanced nursing practice in two countries: An exploratory qualitative comparative study. Nursing Outlook. 2019;**67**(4):365-380. DOI: 10.1016/j.outlook.2019.02.002

[3] Busca E, Savatteri A, Calafato T, Mazzoleni B, Barisone M, Dal Molin A. Barriers and facilitators to the implementation of nurse's role in primary care settings: An integrative review. BMC Nursing. 2021;**20**(1):1-12. DOI: 10.1186/s12912-021-00696-y

[4] Fealy G, Rohde D, Casey M, Brady A, Hegarty J, Kennedy C, et al. Facilitators and barriers in expanding scope of practice: Findings from a national survey of Irish nurses and midwives. Journal of Clinical Nursing. 2015;**24**:3615-3626. DOI: 10.1111/jocn.12980

[5] Nova Scotia College of Nurses. Nursing scope of practice: Practice guideline. 2022. Available from: https://cdn1.nscn.ca/sites/default/files/documents/resources/Scope_of_Practice2020.pdf

[6] Saskatchewan Registered Nurses Association. Nurse practitioner entry-level competencies. 2017. Available from: https://www.crns.ca/nursing-practice/nursing-practice-resources/rnnp-resources/

[7] Verma S, Paterson M, Medves J. Core competencies for health care professionals: What medicine, nursing, occupational therapy, and physiotherapy share. Journal of Allied Health. 2006;**35**(2):109-115

[8] Kaasalainen S, Martin-Misener R, Kilpatrick K, Harbman P, Bryant-Lukosius D, Donald F, et al. A historical overview of the development of advanced nursing practice roles in Canada. Canadian Journal of Nursing Leadership. 2010;**23**:35-60

[9] Canadian Nurses Association. Advanced practice nursing. 2022. Available from: https://www.cna-aiic.ca/en/nursing/advanced-nursing-practice

[10] Canadian Nurses Association. Advanced practice nursing: A pan-Canadian framework. 2019. Available from: https://www.cna-aiic.ca/en/nursing/advanced-nursing-practice

[11] Staples E, Ray S, Hannon R. Canadian Perspectives on Advanced Practice Nursing. Toronto, ON: Canadian Scholars' Press; 2016

[12] Black S, Fadaak R, Myles L. Integrating nurse practitioners into primary care: Policy considerations from a Canadian province. BMC Family Practice. 2020;**21**:254. DOI: 10.1186/s12875-020-01318-3

[13] Marceau R. Sustainability Failures: The Challenge of Sustaining the NP Role and Other Innovations in Primary Health Care. [Unpublished doctoral dissertation]. Edmonton, Canada: University of Alberta; 2020

[14] Stanik-Hutt J, Newhouse R, White K, Johantgen M, Bass E, Zangaro G, et al. The quality and effectiveness of care provided by nurse practitioners. The Journal for Nurse practitioners.

2013;**9**:492-500. DOI: 10.1016/j.nurpra.2013.07.004

[15] Kleinpell RM, Grabenkort WR, Kapu AN, Constantine R, Sicoutris C. Nurse practitioners and physician assistants in acute and critical care: A concise review of the literature and data 2008-2018. Critical Care Medicine. 2019;**47**(10):1442-1449. DOI: 10.1097/CCM.0000000000003925

[16] Canadian Institute of Health Information. Nurse practitioner. 2021. Available from: https://www.cihi.ca/en/nurse-practitioners#:~:text=Key%20findings,with%20other%20regulated%20nursing%20professionals

[17] Archibald M, Fraser K. The potential for nurse practitioners in healthcare reform. Journal of Professional Nursing. 2013;**29**(5):270-275. DOI: 10.1016/j.profnurs.2012.10.002

[18] Kilpatrick K, Lavoie-Tremblay M, Ritchie JA, Lamothe L, Doran D, Rochefort C. How are acute care nurse practitioners enacting their roles in healthcare teams? A descriptive multiple-case study. International Journal of Nursing Studies. 2012;**49**(7):850-862. DOI: 10.1016/j.ijnurstu.2012.01.011

[19] Rickards T, Hamilton S. Patient experiences of primary care provided by nurse practitioners in New Brunswick, Canada. Journal for Nurse Practitioners. 2020;**16**(4):299-304. DOI: 10.1016/j.nurpra.2019.12.027

[20] Sangster-Gormley E, Martin R, Downe-Wamboldt B, Dicenso A. Factors affecting nurse practitioner role implementation in Canadian practice setting: An integrative review. Journal of Advanced Nursing. 2011;**67**(6):1178-1190

[21] Torrens C, Campbell P, Hoskins G, Strachan H, Wells M, Cunningham M, et al. Barriers and facilitators to the implementation of the advanced nurse practitioner role in primary care setting: A scoping review. International Journal of Nursing Studies. 2020;**104**:103443. DOI: 10.1016/j.ijnurstu.2019.103443

[22] Sangster-Gormley E. Prescribing patterns of nurse practitioners in Canada. Canadian Medical Association Journal. 2016;**188**(3):173-174. DOI: 10.1503/cmaj.150913

[23] Canadian Institute for Health Information. Nurse practitioner scopes of practice in Canada. 2021. Available from: https://www.cihi.ca/en/nurse-practitioner-scopes-of-practice-in-canada-2020

[24] Canadian Nurses Protective Society. Medical assistance in dying: What every nurse needs to know. 2021. Available from: https://cnps.ca/article/medical-assistance-in-dying-what-every-nurse-should-know/

[25] Canadian Institute for Health Information. Health workforce in Canada, 2021: Quick stats. 2022. Available from: https://www.cihi.ca/sites/default/files/document/health-workforce-quickstats-2021-data-tables-en.xlsx

[26] Jamison T, Lis G. Engaging the learner by bridging the gap between theory and clinical competence: The impact of concept mapping and simulation as innovative strategies for nurse-sensitive outcomes indicators. Nursing Clinics of North America. 2014;**49**(1):69-80

[27] Benner P. From Novice to Expert: Excellence and Power in Clinical Nursing Practice. Upper Saddle River, NJ: Prentice hall; 2001

[28] Nabizadeh-Gharghozar Z, Alavi N, Ajorpaz N. Clinical competence

in nursing: A hybrid concept analysis. Nurse Education Today. 2021;**94**:104728. DOI: 10.1016/j.nedt.2020.104728

[29] Taylor I, Bing-Jonsson P, Finnbakk E, Wangsteen S, Sandvik L, Fagerstrom L. Development of clinical competence: A longitudinal survey of nurse practitioner students. BMC Nursing. 2021;**20**(1):130-140. DOI: 10.1186/s12912-021-00627-x

[30] Brault I, Kilpatrick K, D'Amour D, ContandriopoulosD,ChouinardV,DuboisCA, et al. Role clarification processes for better integration of nurse practitioners into primary healthcare teams: A multiple-case study. Nursing Research and Practice. 2014;**2014**:1-9. DOI: 10.1155/2014/170514

[31] Nova Scotia College of Nursing. Entry-level competencies for nurse practitioners in Canada adopted by NSCN. 2016. Available from: https://www.nscn.ca/sites/default/files/documents/resources/EntryLevelCompetenciesNP.pdf

[32] Truth and Reconciliation Commission of Canada. Truth and Reconciliation Commission of Canada: Calls to action. 2015. Available from: http://www.trc.ca/websites/trcinstitution/File/2015/Findings/Calls_to_Action_English2.pdf

[33] Bryant-Lukosius D, Carter N, Kilpatrick K, Martin-Misener R, Donald F, Kassalainen S, et al. The clinical nurse specialist role in Canada. Nursing Leadership. 2010;**23**:140-166. DOI: 10.12927/cjnl.2010.22273

[34] Canadian Association of Schools of Nursing. Nurse practitioner education in Canada: Final report. 2011. Available from: https://casn.ca/wp-content/uploads/2014/12/Environmental Scanof NursePractitionerProgramsEn.pdf

[35] Canadian Council of Registered Nurse Regulators. Competencies in the context of entry-level registered nurse practice. 2022. Available from: http://www.ccrnr.ca/entry-to-practice.html

[36] Canadian Council of Registered Nurse Regulators. Practice analysis study of nurse practitioner. 2016. Available from: https://www.ccrnr.ca/assets/ccrnr-practice-analysis-study-of-nurse-practitioners-report---final.pdf

[37] Saskatchewan Registered Nurse Association. Registered nurse (nurse practitioner) entry-level competences. 2017. Available from: https://www.srna.org/wp-content/uploads/2018/01/RNNP-Entry-Level-Competencies-2017.pdf

[38] Alden-Bugden D. The role and scope of the NP in Canada. The Nurse Practitioner. 2019;**44**(9):8-10. DOI: 10.1097/01.NPR.0000577972.50219.34

[39] Canam C. Illuminating the clinical nurse specialist role of advanced practice nursing: A qualitative study. Nursing Leadership. 2005;**18**(4):70-89. DOI: 10.12927/cjnl.2005.17836

[40] Martin-Misener R, Bryant-Lukosius D, Harbman P, Donald F, Kaasalainen S, Carter N, et al. Education of advanced practice nurses in Canada. Nursing Leadership. 2010;**23**:61-84

[41] Canadian Nurses Association. Position statement: Clinical nurse specialist. 2009. Available from: https://hl-prod-ca-oc-download.s3-ca-central-1.amazonaws.com/CNA/2f975e7e-4a40-45ca-863c-5ebf0a138d5e/UploadedImages/documents/Clinical_Nurse_Specialist_position_statement.pdf

[42] Tomblin Murphy G, Sampalli T, Bourque Bearskin L, Cashen N, Cummings A, Elliott Rose A, et al. Investing in Canada's nursing workforce post-pandemic: A call to action. Facets.

2022;**7**(1):1051-1120. DOI: 10.1139/facets-2022-0002

[43] Boamah S, Callen M, Cruz E. Nursing faculty shortage in Canada: A scoping review of contributing factors. Nursing Outlook. 2021;**69**(4):574-588. DOI: 10.1016/j.outlook.2021.01.018

Chapter 4

# Application of Operations Research to Healthcare

*Jia Guo*


## Abstract

Operations research (OR) is significantly important to healthcare. OR techniques can make efficient use of medical resources to enhance patients, providers and agencies' satisfaction. Given limited medical resources and high demand from patients, the primary goal of OR is to use optimization models to quantify the problem and apply mathematical algorithms to obtain a close-to-optimal solution. For example, OR has been widely used to scheduling problems by minimizing the number of nurses or maximizing demand coverage, while keeping service regulations satisfied. In this chapter, we first give a brief introduction of optimization models, followed by the application of OR to healthcare problems such as nurse scheduling, home healthcare delivery and transportation services for patients.


**Keywords:** operations research, mixed integer linear programming, mathematical models, healthcare optimization, nurse scheduling, home healthcare delivery, transportation service

## 1. Introduction

Operations research (OR) plays a critical role in healthcare of both rich and poor countries, especially when the medical resources are limited and the patient demand is high. OR techniques could be applied to optimize the use of medical resources, signicantly improve service quality and reduce operations cost. For example, techniques such as mixed integer linear programming (MILP) algorithms, heuristics and data analytics could be used to design nurse schedules, patient-provider assignment and transportation routes. The past experience has shown that it is possible to obtain high-quality solutions to the most difficult planning and scheduling problems by applying mathematical modeling and advanced decomposition techniques in conjunction with intelligent heuristics.

The general idea of OR application to healthcare is to make decisions by mathematical optimization models. Examples of mathematical formulation on a nurse scheduling problem and a routing problem will be presented in Sections 2 and 3, respectively. Before making decisions, we must have several components that pass on to the optimization model our requirements. Components include:

1. Objective function

    The objective function is the goal we wish to achieve. It can be the minimization of "cost" (such as the number of hired nurses, overtime hours, or patients' travel distance), or the maximization of "profit" (such as hospital revenue, patient demand coverage, or satisfaction level). Some problems require a multi-objective function. For example, hospitals aim to achieve maximum patient demand coverage with a minimum number of nurses.

2. Constraints

    Constraints are the rules and regulations we must obey. For example, nurses cannot work 20 hours a day, even though the violation of this rule can cover more patient demand with fewer nurses. Constraints that cannot be violated are considered "hard." In addition to hard constraints, there are "soft" constraints that can be violated with a penalty cost added to the objective function. For instance, nurses are not encouraged to work more than 40 hours per week, but overtime is allowed if all the demands must be covered. If a nurse works overtime for an hour, then the one-hour penalty cost is added to the objective function. That means all demand is covered at the cost of overtime.

3. Decision variables

    Decision variables indicate what we are supposed to decide. For example, in a home healthcare delivery problem, we need to decide on nurse-patient assignment, nurses' travel routes, and service start time at each patient's location.

4. Parameters

    Parameters are given as constants. For instance, when designing nurses' travel routes, we know the distance between every two locations. In real-life problems, however, some parameters are uncertain, such as patient demand and travel time, which may vary during different periods of the day. In such cases, robust optimization will be involved to address uncertainty.

In practical cases, a mathematical optimization model usually contains thousands, even tens and thousands of decision variables, making it extremely time-consuming for commercial solvers (such as CPLEX or Gurobi) to get a good solution within a reasonable amount of time. In reality, a lot of health institutes are reluctant to purchase the license of commercial solvers due to the high price. Therefore, mathematical algorithms (optimization-based heuristics or metaheuristics) are developed to solve large-scale problems. Optimization-based algorithms usually require solutions to mathematical models, but instead of solving the large-scale problem directly, the problem can be decomposed or transferred to smaller and easier problems. Common optimization-based algorithms include but are not limited to Lagrangian Relaxation, Column Generation, Benders Decomposition, Cutting Plane Algorithm and so forth. Metaheuristics do not rely on the type of the problem, but it must keep all the hard constraints satisfied while searching for a close-to-optimal solution. Metaheuristics include but are not limited to Genetic Algorithm, Greedy Algorithm, Tabu Search, Ant Colony Algorithm, Simulated Annealing, and Memetic Algorithm. Even though optimization-based algorithms and metaheuristics can find good feasible solutions within a limited amount of time, they are both at the cost of optimality. The quality of solutions obtained from the algorithm significantly depends on the algorithm parameters, such as time limit and the number of iterations for each step.

The remainder of this chapter displays several examples of OR application to healthcare, such as nurse scheduling, home healthcare delivery, and transportation services for patients.

## 2. Nurse scheduling

Nurse scheduling is a critical branch of OR application to healthcare. Nurses are of vital essence in hospital and clinic operations, generally accounting for more than 50% of the budget [1]. The efficient use of nursing resources can directly impact a healthcare system's financial well-being. This is true for both public and private facilities, and especially true for those that serve economically disadvantaged areas [2].

### 2.1 Problem description

In a nurse scheduling problem, the goal is to assign nurses to different shifts over a one-or-several-week planning horizon. A shift usually lasts 6–12 hours with a fixed start and end time. For example, the start and end time of the morning, evening, and night shifts are (7 am, 3 pm), (3 pm, 11 pm), (11 pm, 7 am), respectively. The union of all shifts covers the entire planning horizon.

The stakeholders in a nurse scheduling problem include nurses and patients. On the side of patients, the demand should be covered as much as possible. That means a sufficient number of nurses should be assigned to each shift, so that patients can receive necessary medical treatment. Also, nurses' skill qualification is of vital significance. For example, a nurse for a blood test cannot be assigned to help a patient with her physical therapy.

On the side of nurses, the laws and regulations are mostly on hours of service. For example, for each nurse, there is an upper and lower limit on the number of working hours and working days per week, the number of consecutive working days and days off, the number of consecutive working hours, the number of overtime hours per week, the number of shifts per day, and the number of weekend shifts. In addition, each nurse must rest for at least 8 hours between any two shifts assigned to her.

Furthermore, some clinics and hospitals allow nurses to report on their preference for days and shifts before the schedule is decided. For example, if a nurse reports her preferred working day is Sep. 28, and she will not be available on Oct. 1, then a "profit" will be added to the objective function if a shift is assigned on Sep. 28, and a "cost" will be incurred if she is scheduled to work on Oct. 1. Other factors contributing to nurses' satisfaction level include shift transition, work-day transition, and equity. The shift transition happens if a nurse is assigned different shifts on two consecutive days (e.g., morning shift on day 1 and evening shift on day 2). Shift transition makes it harder for nurses to keep a regular life schedule. Work-day transition involves two cases: (i) 1-0-1 schedule: work on day 1, rest on day 2, work on day 3; and (ii) 0-1-0 schedule: rest on day 1, work on day 2, rest on day 3. Neither 1-0-1 nor 0-1-0 schedule is beneficial as they add an interruption to nurses' work or rest. Equity means the number of overtime hours, 1-0-1 schedules, 0-1-0 schedules, or any other preference violations should be evenly spread among nurses. For example, it is not ideal to assign nurse A 20-hour overtime, while asking nurse B not to work overtime at all.

## 2.2 Mathematical optimization model

The requirements for nurses and patients can be either "soft" or "hard" constraints, depending on the hospital or legal regulations. In this subsection, a mathematical formulation for the nurse scheduling problem (Model 1) is presented. For simplicity, we assume the planning horizon is 1 week. The objective function is to minimize the number of uncovered demand hours, 1-0-1 violations, 0-1-0 violations, and violation differences among nurses. The hard constraints include the upper and lower limits on the number of working hours for each nurse in a week. Each nurse can work at most one shift per day.

*Sets and indices*

| | |
|---|---|
| $a$ | index for 1-0-1 or 0-1-0 schedule violation $a$ |
| $d$ | index for day $d$ |
| $h$ | index for hour $h$ |
| $i$ | index for nurse $i$ |
| $t$ | index for shift $t$ |
| $D$ | set of days in the planning horizon |
| $H$ | set of hours on each day |
| $LD_n$ | last $n$ days of the planning horizon being scheduled |
| $N$ | set of nurses |
| $T$ | set of shifts |

*Parameters*

| | |
|---|---|
| $\alpha$ | weight for an uncovered demand, assuming weight for 1-0-1 and 0-1-0 violation is 1 |
| $D_{dh}$ | demand (the number of nurses required) in hour $h$ on day $d$ |
| $F_{ht}$ | 1 if shift $t$ covers hour $h$, 0 otherwise |
| $\overline{H}_i, \underline{H}_i$ | the upper and lower limits of the number of working hours for each nurse during the planning horizon |
| $h_t$ | the length of shift $t$, which is the difference between start and end time of shift $t$ |
| $r_a$ | penalty for $a$ violations, $a = 1, 2, \ldots, V_{\max}$ |
| $V_{\max}$ | maximum number of preference violations allowed for each nurse |

*Decision variables*

| | |
|---|---|
| $P_{id}$ | (accounting) 1 if nurse $i$ has a 0-1-0 pattern schedule starting on day $d$, 0 otherwise |
| $Q_{id}$ | (accounting) 1 if nurse $i$ has a 1-0-1 pattern schedule starting on day $d$, 0 otherwise |
| $U_{dh}$ | uncovered demand on day $d$ in hour $h$ |
| $V_{ia}$ | (binary) 1 if nurse $i$ has $a$ violations, 0 otherwise |
| $X_{idt}$ | (binary) 1 if nurse $i$ is assigned to shift $t$ on day $d$, 0 otherwise |

Model 1

$$\text{Minimize} \quad \alpha \sum_{d\in D}\sum_{h\in H} U_{dh} + \sum_{i\in N}\sum_{a=1}^{V_{\max}} r_a V_{ia} \tag{1}$$

subject to

1. Demand constraints

$$U_{dh} \geq D_{dh} - \sum_{i\in N}\sum_{t\in T} F_{ht} X_{idt} \qquad \forall\ h\in H,\ \ d\in D \tag{2}$$

2. Upper and lower limits on the number of working hours for each nurse in the planning horizon

$$\sum_{d\in D}\sum_{t\in T} h_t X_{idt} \leq \overline{H}_i \qquad \forall\ i\in N \tag{3}$$

$$\sum_{d\in D}\sum_{t\in T} h_t X_{idt} \geq \underline{H}_i \qquad \forall\ i\in N \tag{4}$$

3. At most one shift per day for each nurse

$$\sum_{t\in T} X_{idt} \leq 1 \qquad \forall\ i\in N,\ \ d\in D \tag{5}$$

4. Definition of 0-1-0 and 1-0-1 violations

$$\sum_{t\in T} X_{idt} + \left(1 - \sum_{t\in T} X_{i,d+1,t}\right) + \sum_{t\in T} X_{i,d+2,t} + P_{id} \geq 1 \qquad \forall\ d\in D\backslash LD_2,\ \ i\in N \tag{6}$$

$$\left(1 - \sum_{t\in T} X_{idt}\right) + \sum_{t\in T} X_{i,d+1,t} + \left(1 - \sum_{t\in T} X_{i,d+2,t}\right) + Q_{id} \geq 1 \qquad \forall\ d\in D\backslash LD_2, i\in N \tag{7}$$

5. Violation computation

$$\sum_{d\in D} (P_{id} + Q_{id}) = \sum_{a=1}^{V_{\max}} a V_{ia} \qquad \forall\ i\in N \tag{8}$$

6. Variables definition

$$X_{idt},\ \ P_{id},\ \ Q_{id},\ \ V_{ia} \in \{0,1\} \qquad \forall\ i\in N,\ \ d\in D,\ \ t\in T,\ \ 0\leq a\leq V_{\max} \tag{9}$$

$$0 \leq U_{dh} \leq D_{dh} \qquad \forall\ d\in D,\ \ h\in H \tag{10}$$

Objective function (1) consists of two terms. The first term is the weighted demand uncoverage, that is, sum of the number of nurses required but not supplied in each hour every day. If the hospital requires 10 nurses on Monday between 8:00 am and 9:00 am, but only 7 nurses are assigned to this hour, then we have uncovered a demand of 3, that is, $U_{\text{Mon},8} = 3$. Instead of adding 3 directly to the objective function, we add $3\alpha$ to quantify the significance of demand coverage. The weight for an uncovered demand ($\alpha$) is usually larger than 1 because we give demand coverage a higher priority. The second term is the penalty for 1-0-1 and 0-1-0 violations. Binary variable $V_{ia} = 1$ if nurse $i$ has $a$ 1-0-1 and 0-1-0 violations throughout the planning horizon. Note that $r_a$ is usually a constant exponential of $a$. For example, if nurse $i$ has 3 1-0-1 and 0-1-0 violations, then a penalty cost of $e^3$ will be added to the objective function. We use a constant exponential of $a$ because we would like to improve equity among nurses, that is, not to assign one particular nurse a large number of violations, while giving other nurses few violations.

Constraints (2) define the number of uncovered demands in each hour every day. On the right-hand side of (2), $D_{dh}$ is the number of nurses required in hour $h$ on day $d$. The term $\sum_{i\in N}\sum_{t\in T} F_{ht}X_{idt}$ indicates the number of nurses scheduled to work in hour $h$ on day $d$. We use "$\geq$" instead of "$=$" in this set of constraints due to the following reasons:

1. If $D_{dh} - \sum_{i\in N}\sum_{t\in T} F_{ht}X_{idt} \geq 0$, then there is no over-coverage in hour $h$ on day $d$. Even though constraints (2) require the variable $U_{dh}$ to be greater than or equal to $D_{dh} - \sum_{i\in N}\sum_{t\in T} F_{ht}X_{idt}$, the objective function automatically makes $U_{dh} = D_{dh} - \sum_{i\in N}\sum_{t\in T} F_{ht}X_{idt}$ due to its nature of minimization.

2. If $D_{dh} - \sum_{i\in N}\sum_{t\in T} F_{ht}X_{idt} < 0$, then there is over-coverage in hour $h$ on day $d$. Since variable $U_{dh}$ is defined to be nonnegative, $U_{dh} = 0$.

Constraints (3) and (4) force each nurse to work between $\underline{H}_i$ and $\overline{H}_i$ hours in the planning horizon. Constraints (5) require a nurse should work at most one shift per day. Constraints (6) and (7) indicate whether nurse $i$ has a 0-1-0 or 1-0-1 violation starting on day $d$. Take constraints (6) for example, if nurse $i$ rests on day $d$ (i.e., $\sum_{t\in T} X_{idt} = 0$), works on day $d + 1$ (i.e., $\sum_{t\in T} X_{i,d+1,t} = 1$) and rests on day $d + 2$ (i.e., $\sum_{t\in T} X_{i,d+2,t} = 0$), then to make constraint (6) satisfied, binary variable $P_{id}$ must equal 1, indicating nurse $i$ has a 0-1-0 violation starting on day $d$. Constraints (8) calculate the total number of 0-1-0 and 1-0-1 violations. Constraints (9) and (10) give variables definitions.

## 3. Home healthcare delivery

Home healthcare (HHC) delivery plays an important role in medical service, especially for patients with chronic illnesses and ambulatory disabilities. Instead of requiring patients to travel to hospital for medical treatment, hospitals schedule qualified nurses to provide service for patients at their place of residence. The quality of the weekly and daily schedules assigned to the nurses can impact the level of service patients receive, as well as nurse productivity and job satisfaction. Efficient patient-nurse scheduling and routing can significantly reduce the cost and improve the service quality of HHC.

### 3.1 Problem description

In a home healthcare scheduling and routing (HHCSR) problem, nurses are scheduled to provide medical treatment for patients who reside in different locations of a city. On each day of the planning horizon, a nurse starts from home (or a depot), visits patients that are assigned to her, and returns home. Decision variables include (i) nurse-patient assignment, that is, which nurse should be assigned to visit each patient; (ii) the travel route of each nurse (i.e., visit sequence of patients for each nurse); and (iii) nurses' arrival time at patients' home. The objective of an HHCSR problem includes but is not limited to the minimization of nurses' travel distance and the maximization of patients' satisfaction level. Details of each stakeholder will be discussed in the remainder of this subsection.

#### *3.1.1 Patients*

Before the agency (clinic or hospital) designs nurses' assignments and routes, patients request visits with specific service dates, time windows, and skill requirements. Nurses' schedules and routes are designed based on the information from patients. In addition to meeting the requirements on time and skill qualification, the agency should try to keep the continuity of care (CoC) for patients with multiple visits in the planning horizon by assigning the same nurse to a patient. CoC has the benefit of maintaining treatment consistency as the nurse becomes more familiar with the patient's physical condition and treatment details.

#### *3.1.2 Nurses*

To ensure the nurses can provide high-quality service for patients, the daily workload of each nurse is limited to a specified range. The workload can be associated with the number of working hours, the number of patients serviced, and the type of medical treatment offered by the nurse. In addition, nurses usually have agreements with the agency on the start and end time of each day. However, in some cases, nurses are allowed to work overtime to complete more requested visits. Moreover, the differences in workload among nurses with the same skill level should be minimized to achieve the objective of equity. Finally, to provide a healthy working environment, a lunch break is taken into account.

The requirements from patients and nurses can be either "hard" or "soft" constraints in the optimization problem, depending on the agreement among patients, nurses, and the agency. If a constraint is relaxed as a "soft" constraint and is violated in a schedule, then we should add a penalty cost to the objective function.

The above paragraphs describe the basic version of a HHCSR problem. In practice, the problem can be extended and involve more stakeholders. For example, in some cases, on each day of the planning horizon, nurses start from pharmacies, visit patients to drop off medicine, provide medical treatment, and collect biological samples (such as blood or tissue). After visiting all the scheduled patients, nurses deliver all collected biological samples to laboratories for tests [3]. In such cases, besides decisions in the basic version of a HHCSR problem, patient-pharmacy assignment and pharmacy-laboratory assignment should be made. Furthermore, vehicle capacity must be considered due to the transportation of medicine and biological samples.

### 3.2 Mathematical optimization model

In this subsection, we assume the nurse-patient assignment is completed by clustering based on the geographical locations of patients. Model 2 decides the sequence of requested visits assigned to nurse $w$ on day $d$, as well as the service start time of each visit. The objective is to minimize the travel time, the number of hours a visit is completed outside of the patient's time window, and the number of hours nurse $w$ works overtime. Model 2 makes use of following notation.

*Sets and indices*

| | |
|---|---|
| $i$ | index for requested visit |
| $I_{dw}$ | set of all requested visits to be completed by nurse $w$ on day $d$ |

*Parameters*

| | |
|---|---|
| $\alpha$ | penalty weight of travel time in the objective function |
| $h^{s}_{dw}, h^{e}_{dw}$ | start and end time of nurse $w$'s shift on day $d$ |
| $h^{s}_{i}, h^{e}_{i}$ | start and end time of the time window for requested visit $i$ |
| $t_i$ | service time for visit $i$; amount of time nurse $w$ spends on visit $i$ excluding travel time |
| $\tau_{ii'}$ | travel time from the location of requested visit $i$ to that of $i'$ |

*Decision variables*

| | |
|---|---|
| $T_{diw}$ | (continuous) time when nurse $w$ begins treatment for visit $i$ on day $d$ |
| $X_{dii'w}$ | (binary) 1 if visit $i'$ is scheduled immediately after visit $i$ for nurse $w$ on day $d$, 0 otherwise |
| $Y^{VS}_{diw}, Y^{VE}_{diw}$ | (continuous) length of time window violation for an early or late arrival of nurse $w$ for visit $i$ on day $d$ |
| $Y^{WS}_{diw}, Y^{WE}_{diw}$ | (continuous) number of hours outside of the start or end time of a shift for nurse $w$ on visit $i$ on day $d$ |

Model 2 (for fixed nurse $w$ on day $d$)

$$\text{Minimize} \quad \alpha \sum_{i \in I_{dw}} \sum_{i' \in I_{dw}} \tau_{ii'} X_{dii'w} + \sum_{i \in I_{dw}} \left( Y^{VS}_{diw} + Y^{VE}_{diw} + Y^{WS}_{diw} + Y^{WE}_{diw} \right) \tag{11}$$

subject to.
Each visit has a predecessor and successor on a route

$$\sum_{i' \in I_{dw}} X_{dii'w} = 1 \qquad \forall\ i \in I_{dw} \tag{12}$$

$$\sum_{i \in I_{dw}} X_{dii'w} = 1 \qquad \forall\ i' \in I_{dw} \tag{13}$$

Violation of patient time windows

$$Y_{diw}^{\mathrm{VS}} \geq h_i^{\mathrm{s}} - T_{diw} \qquad \forall\ i \in I_{dw} \tag{14}$$

$$Y_{diw}^{\mathrm{VE}} \geq T_{diw} + t_i - h_i^{\mathrm{e}} \qquad \forall\ i \in I_{dw} \tag{15}$$

Violation of shift start and end times

$$Y_{diw}^{\mathrm{WS}} \geq h_{dw}^{\mathrm{s}} - T_{diw} \qquad \forall\ i \in I_{dw} \tag{16}$$

$$Y_{diw}^{\mathrm{WE}} \geq T_{diw} + t_i - h_{dw}^{\mathrm{e}} \qquad \forall\ i \in I_{dw} \tag{17}$$

Subtour elimination constraints

$$T_{diw} + (\tau_{ii'} + t_i) - M(1 - X_{dii'w}) \leq T_{di'w} \qquad \forall\ i \neq i' \in I_{dw} \tag{18}$$

Variables definitions

$$X_{dii'w} \in \{0, 1\} \qquad \forall\ i \neq i' \in I_{dw} \tag{19}$$

$$Y_{diw}^{\mathrm{VS}},\ Y_{diw}^{\mathrm{VE}},\ Y_{diw}^{\mathrm{WS}},\ Y_{diw}^{\mathrm{WE}} \geq 0 \qquad \forall\ i \in I_{dw} \tag{20}$$

$$T_{diw} \geq 0 \qquad \forall\ i \in I_{dw} \tag{21}$$

Objective function (11) contains two terms. The first term minimizes the travel time. The second term minimizes four components. The first two components represent the length of time window violation for an early or late arrival of nurse $w$ for visit $i$ on day $d$. The third and fourth components are the number of hours outside of the start or end time of a shift for nurse $w$ on day $d$.

Constraints (12) and (13) ensure that each requested visit has exactly one predecessor and successor on a route, assuming there is a dummy origin and destination. This makes the route a closed loop. Constraints (14) and (15) calculate the number of hours a visit is completed outside of its time window. Constraints (16) and (17) compute the number of hours nurse $w$ works overtime. Constraints (18) prevent the model from creating subtours among the requested visit locations. Constraints (19)–(21) define the variables range.

## 4. Transportation services for patients

Transportation services for nonemergency medical appointments are of vital importance, especially to financially disadvantaged patients. In urban communities, a lot of poor patients cannot afford a car, and thus they have to rely on public transportation to keep medical appointments. However, public transportation is insufficient and inconvenient for people with ambulatory issues. As a result, clinics experience high cancelation/no-show rates. Moreover, many patients do not have the means to pick up their medicine after appointments, which makes their situation even worse. Good transportation services can significantly help patients to keep appointments and save operations costs of the clinic [4].

Unlike the problem described in Sections 2 and 3, offering transportation services for patients can hardly be integrated into one single optimization model but involves multiple problems such as the prediction of no-show rate, the decision on transportation mode, and the assignment of transportation services. The remainder of this subsection introduces details of each problem.

### 4.1 Prediction of no-show probability

When designing transportation services for patients with nonemergency medical appointments, we first need to investigate the impact of transportation barriers on no-show, and predict the no-show probability assuming the transportation service is not available. This can be achieved by collecting patients' historical data, such as home address, transportation difficulty level, transportation mode, ambulatory issue, and travel time, whether they have chronic diseases, and whether they kept their appointments. Then, statistical analysis can be conducted to predict the no-show probability based on those factors, and verify whether the transportation barrier significantly impacts the no-show probability. Logistic regression models can be applied to predict the probability. This step shows whether providing transportation services is necessary, and recognizes the group of patients that need transportation services [5, 6].

### 4.2 Decision on transportation mode

Unlike regular urban transportation, transportation services for patients must be uniquely designed due to patients' weak physical conditions. Therefore, the transportation mode should meet the following requirements. First, the transportation mode should allow patients to either sit or stand. For example, it is improper to offer free bicycles to patients. Second, some patients have ambulatory issues, so the transportation mode must have enough capacity to hold wheelchairs. Third, some clinics or hospitals do not have bus stations nearby, so the transportation service should give patients a ride to their destination. Finally, the transportation mode should allow patients to receive service without long waiting, especially in areas of severe weather. Based on the above requirements, taxis and shuttle buses with short intervals are common transportation services provided for patients.

### 4.3 Vehicle routing-based optimization problem

The vehicle routing-based optimization problem is a crucial branch of transportation services if shuttle buses are offered. In a regular vehicle routing problem, vehicles depart from a depot, visit several locations and return to the depot. In a medical situation for patients, each vehicle starts from the clinic, visits several stops to pick up and drop off patients, and goes back to the clinic. In this optimization problem, we need to decide the number of vehicles, the route of each vehicle, and the vehicle's arrival time at each stop. With a rough estimation of the number of patients at each bus stop, we should also take vehicle capacity into consideration. Moreover, the shuttle interval and travel time must be restricted to an upper bound for the sake of patients' health conditions. The objective can be minimization of vehicles' fixed cost, travel cost, patients' waiting, or travel time. Examples of vehicle routing problem models can be found in Luo et al. [7] and Guo et al. [4].

## 5. Summary

Operations research has been widely applied to healthcare by maximizing the benefits of all stakeholders with a limited amount of medical resources. In addition to nurse scheduling, home healthcare delivery, and transportation services for patients, other problems such as operating room and surgeon assignment, inventory management of medical material, and healthcare project prioritization can also be addressed by mathematical models and algorithms.

Besides knowledge and skills in healthcare management, mathematics, and computer, expertise in other fields plays a crucial role in OR application. For example, topology and network theories are of vital importance in transportation design, and inventory techniques can significantly improve the order and storage decisions of medical material. The OR application to healthcare is a combination of mathematics, computer skills, medical knowledge, and a variety of interdisciplinary expertise.

## Author details

Jia Guo
Operations Research and Industrial Engineering, Cockrell School of Engineering, The University of Texas, Austin, TX, United States of America

*Address all correspondence to: jia.guo@utexas.edu

## References

[1] Chiang B. Estimating nursing costs—A methodological review. International Journal of Nursing Studies. 2009;**46**(5): 716-722

[2] Guo J, Bard JF. A column generation-based algorithm for midterm nurse scheduling with specialized constraints, preference considerations, and overtime. Computers and Operations Research. 2022;**138**(2022):105597. DOI: 10.1016/j.cor.2021.105597

[3] Bahadori-Chinibelagh S, Fathollahi-Fard AM, Hajiaghaei-Keshteli M. Two constructive algorithms to address a multi-depot home healthcare routing problem. IETE Journal of Research. 2019;**68**(3):1-7. DOI: 10.1080/03772063.2019.1642802

[4] Guo J, Bard JF, Morrice DJ, Jaén CR, Poursani R. Offering transportation services to economically disadvantaged patients at a family health center: A case study. Health Systems. 2022;**11**(4): 251-275

[5] Mohammadi I, Wu H, Turkcan A, Toscos T, Doebbeling BN. Data analytics and modeling for appointment No-show in community health centers. Journal of Primary Care & Community Health. 2018;**9**:1-11

[6] Topuz K, Uner H, Oztekin A, Yildirim MB. Predicting pediatric clinic no-shows: A decision analytic framework using elastic net and Bayesian belief network. Annals of Operations Research. 2018;**263**(1–2): 479-499

[7] Luo Z, Liu M, Lim A. A two-phase branch-and-price-and-cut for a dial-a-ride problem in patient transportation. Transportation Science. 2019;**53**(1): 113-130

Chapter 5

# Nurse Practitioners "Insider" and "Outsider" Roles and Responsibilities Enabling a Quality Managed Delivery of Contemporary Medical Imaging Services

*Chandra Rekha Makanjee*


## Abstract

Nurse practitioners (NPs), as key healthcare professional, play a critical role in the provision and coordination of care, prevention of adverse events, health service throughput, and patient outcomes. Patient experience is considered as one of the pillars of quality in healthcare, along with patient safety and clinical outcomes. Based on the aforementioned, nurse practitioners have a vital role in providing clinical nursing care to patients within or outside of the immediate medical imaging (MI) working environment. Their evolving role expansion in medical imaging is documented in the literature. The purpose of this chapter is to create further awareness of the nurse practitioner in medical imaging.


**Keywords:** quality, management, contemporary, services delivery, nurses

## 1. Introduction

In health care organizations, nurse practitioners (NP) play a pivotal role in serving as a liaison between multi disciplines including the temporary team membership in medical imaging (MI) enabling patient care management that strives to achieve consistent, high-quality care [1]. The principle of quality is implicit in healthcare and includes aspects of accessibility, appropriateness, affordability, availability, effectivity, efficiency, integratedness, and safety [2]. Additionally, the continuity of care and wellbeing concept which goes beyond the healthcare complex is essential. Continuity is conceptualized as multidimensional, encompassing three specific domains—relational, management, and informational continuity—with emphasis placed on their interrelations. Continuity of care (CoC) is an important aspect of quality, safety and efficient manner. CoC implies the delivery of services in a coherent, logical, and timely fashion [3]. These NPs form an integral part in the continuity and holistic care using the nursing process of assessment, diagnosis, planning, implementation, and evaluation. Including nursing care to individuals' families, communities, or populations by using critical thinking, skill, professional competence, and evidence-based knowledge.

MI technology is a healthcare resource intertwined and shared across the multilayered healthcare delivery, medical specialties, and patient care. Their services are crucial in the management of various diseases contributing toward CoC, ranging from primary prevention, timely detection, and diagnosis to treatment and post-therapy rehabilitation or palliative care and as well as for fluoroscopic real-time visualization of different types of pathology and image-guided diagnostic tumor sampling for pathology work-up and therapeutic interventions. It aligns with the recent endeavor on the role of medical imaging in value-based healthcare. Including the timely diagnosis highly reliant on the accessibility, effectiveness, efficiency in utilization of the imaging technology [4, 5]. It consists of both ionizing and non-ionizing imaging modalities. The ionizing modalities are general radiography, fluoroscopic imaging examinations, mobile radiography, portable radiography, mammography, computed tomography, angiographic and interventional angiographic imaging examinations, diagnostic nuclear medicine whereas non-ionizing imaging modalities include diagnostic ultrasound and magnetic resonance imaging. The different examination types with its respective imaging modalities and the interpretation of the imaging series are used to diagnose, monitor, or treat medical conditions [4, 6]. From an NP perspective technology form an integral part of the nursing profession and it is expected of them to have that specialized knowledge and insight to recognize, prevent and care for possible complications related to MI examination types [7].

The purpose of the chapter is to provide a bird's eye view of the roles and responsibilities of the NP in MI as an "insider" and "outsider" as the patient journeys through the various points within the healthcare system.

## 2. The nurse practitioner's scope of practice and diagnostic decision-making processes

Quality of care improvement within a healthcare team differs in terms of education, expertise, and competencies. For example, a rich mix of qualified staff with postgraduate qualifications is associated with better clinical outcomes. Globally, there is a widening gap between the supply and demand of healthcare workers indicating a need for an urgent response. Within the bigger picture at the global level bridging, this gap is complex and complicated. Several factors impact the balance of demand and the supply of timely and appropriate care. Within this context, the number of healthcare professionals is only one aspect impacting access to care. In this regard, NPs are positioned in settings such as government roles, public health, academia, clinical care, leadership, and private industries with the ability to develop a creative and effective network to respond to multifaceted problems. Dynamic NPs practicing to its full scope can assist in addressing health system demands [8].

Before this can occur, a clearer understanding and national application of the NP scope of practice is required [9]. Any ambiguity surrounding the practice scope of NP impacts the profession's ability to respond to health system challenges. NP scope of practice is defined and regulated among others by their education, training, clinical experience, registration standards, endorsements and notations, positions of employment, clinical protocols, and guidelines. Efforts to recognize new professions or modify the scope of practice for existing health professions usually require the enactment of or amendment to state law, a process that is typically slow and, at times, adversarial. For example, in the United States of America, states often solicit input on proposed changes from stakeholders, including professional associations and, to a more limited extent, consumer groups [10]. According to Gleason et al. the scope of practice laws is not the barrier as perceived to be [11]. These authors advocate that NPs to be prepared and accountable for playing an active role in the diagnostic process, not that they assume accountability for making medical diagnoses. However, a challenge is a false perception that scope of practice laws prohibits NPs from participating in the diagnostic process. The lack of consistency across states' scope of practice laws and terminology used to describe the role of NPs in medical diagnosis could contribute to the confusion. Therefore, encouraged to adopt clear and common regulatory language that contributes to the medical diagnostic process, is within the NPs scope of practice [11].

However, the reality is that these professionals significantly contribute to the medical diagnostic process, in terms of observations, diagnostic thinking, clinical judgment, reasoning, and interpretations of findings. Gleason and others believe that NPs are essential members of the diagnostic team. Though there is a clinical medical diagnosis by medical healthcare professionals assigned based on a syndrome or disease based on a set of signs, symptoms, and other findings. One could argue that a nursing diagnosis is based on a clinical judgment based on a holistic approach not only isolated to their health conditions but expands beyond the immediate clinical context including family members and community. However, these practitioners also function in acute, chronic, and high-pressure critical medical environments and expectation to identify and intervene through an action plan. This process of diagnostic decision-making encounters includes diagnostic tests like medical imaging encounters that NPs are directly or indirectly involved [11].

From a MI quality management perspective, MI service refers to an understanding of the importance of quality as a determining factor in competitiveness such as globalization, technological evolution, increased competition, changes in the profile of patients in these services [5]. Like any health service, it is an open system and suffers the action of the environment that constantly changes, while it contributed to the emergence of a new way of seeing its internal and external relations to meet new demands of imaging service. Quality of services that occupy an important place in health care is imbued to seek excellence and sustainable development with a focus on risk management, quality of exams, reports, and patient safety improvements [12]. Nursing influences and adds value to the practice in radiology and imaging diagnosis by incorporating assessment skills and initiatives of evidence-based practices, and the nurses' specialization in MI is recognized. Disseminating this specialty and producing knowledge, as well as the methodology of nursing accreditation in this space, require attention, as they are associated with the redefinition of the roles of NPs and other members of the health team [6].

The quality of service regarding the CoC for instance includes on-MI NPs who are responsible for the handoffs and safe transition of patients between inpatient wards and MI departments. CoC occurs through verbal and written reports. That CoC was disrupted because of breakdowns in verbal and written communication. In a study by Carley and others several participants echoed the limited communication about what happened in the MI procedure during handoff. Information shared verbally between the sending and receiving nurses varied. To overcome this shortcoming, a suggestion was to focus on the specifics about the procedure when interacting with medical imaging NPs [13].

## 3. Nurse practitioner referrer and medical image interpreter role

MI studies usually come from referring clinicians during a medical encounter who seek radiological input, and directly receive the output (reports). Referring clinicians can be considered as "intermediate customers". Similarly, it is not unusual for NPs to complete a request order, initiate an imaging referral, varying from country to country. For example, within an Australian primary healthcare context, NPs scope is limited to completing referrals for chest and pelvis radiographic examinations. Restrictions also apply to other imaging examinations such as Dopplers and Dexa scans. These are essential for NPs to be able to access if they are to provide appropriate primary health care and address often urgent health needs without the delay. For example, there are legislative changes proposed by the Australian Capital Territory Government with regard registered NP registered by the Nursing and Midwifery Board of Australia with regard to advanced practice. Like working independently and collaboratively within the ambit of expert critical care context. Includes among other like core activities, such as diagnosis and treatment of medical conditions, prescribing medicine and requesting and interpreting diagnostic examinations (e.g., blood tests and MI examinations) [14].

One of the arguments is the fear of over or under diagnostic tests that would or would not have been ordered by the medical officer. Though the potential benefits of NPs in terms of saving time and satisfaction, there are also excessive requests that could potentially result in additional time, additional expense and increased resource utilization, unnecessary radiation exposure, and potential morbidity. Risk of additional tests following the physician's examination. Additional projections of the same/adjacent or different regions can be ordered because the first projection did not demonstrate the problem, or another injury was discovered during the consultation. The "to and froing" like unnecessary trips to imaging become necessary, resulting in both the time constraints for treatment and the inconvenience to the patient [15, 16].

The request order is an effective and efficient medium of communication between the refer and the recipient on behalf of the patient. The request order is an essential part of the justification for the examination, a medico-legal requirement, provides the cue for the type of MI examination through verification and confirmation with the patient, the planning of the MI examination, compiling a radiological interpretation and report triggering an action plan and form part of the medical record keeping. For example, often MI services are rendered outside of the immediate MI section, such as intensive care units, emergency and trauma settings, and ward settings. In these instances, the justification expands beyond the imaging justification principle. These requests ideally are restricted to patients on life-support machines or those with medical conditions where nursing care and treatment could be seriously affected if transported to the imaging section. If the examination requested could be done in the MI section with a better outcome, the MI team should consult the referring doctor and nurse looking after the patient regarding the advisability of moving [17]. In other words, the referring doctor should always consent to any changes to the mobile imaging service requested. A chore in the element is quality of the information and processing the referral in a timely manner in achieving a high impact quality MI outcome. Bearing in mind that multiple patients and patient acuity levels can prevent the attentiveness needed to process orders in a timely manner. A good working relationship between the doctor, radiographer, and nurse is cardinal in acquiring quality diagnostic images [18].

In most instances, the refer could make a request electronically through the radiology information system (RIS) or paper-based and especially in an emergency by telephone and or bleep system. Digital patient records enable and ensures seamless communication between the departments. If this record is not available and configured in a way that the MI professionals can access and utilize. Inaccessibility and timely access could result in errors, impact safety, compromise the quality of examination, accuracy of results, or potential for delays. It is essential for NPs as referrers to liaise with all involved parties in establishing the information that should be shared at this stage. For example, documenting not only the presence of an intravenous line but also the size of the line can be essential information for MI sections like contrast media-related imaging examinations. Considerable time can be lost if MI staff must track down the referring NP to find out if an intravenous line is capable of the high flow required for some intravenous MI contrast agents.

With modern MI computer science and technological advancement, a chore component of clinical practical applications such as medical diagnosis, treatment planning, and for instance surgical navigation [17, 19]. Including a wide array of technological networks among other social media and e-health data use has resulted in a massive progression in the way MI services are delivered [20]. An essential element throughout these processes is the filtration of the quality documented information in the delivery of quality, evidence-based nursing practice. Since NPs accountability, roles, and responsibilities expand across settings from the micro-level clinical bedside to an administrative office role at the meso and or macro level in an organization. According to Zadvinskis et al., and Abuzaid and others recognise the value of artificial intelligence (AI), like health information system, electronic health records; and digitised order entry and decision aid support in medical imaging and robotics. These cognitive technologies are less invasive and more accurate tools for diagnosis and treatment. The recommendations are for organizations to invest in these technologies, refine the policies and align with nursing practice and integration into nursing education and professional development [21, 22]. Clinical data provide a holistic and collaborative understanding of the clinical condition and the management of patient care. Digital management systems can be of value in terms of data storage which can be transformed into stored electronic clinical data for utilization to provide safe and effective patient care. The design of these clinical systems should address workflow and must be done on a continuous and iterative approach based on identified needs. Good record-keeping is an integral part of patient care. Documentation should extend beyond the confines of the diagnostic report. An integrated "event details" section would allow important information to be recorded through an integrated clinical environment platform. As part of the patient clinical notes and discharge summary, thus reducing the risk of conflicting information between patient information held on the RIS and information in the patient notes. Thereby, maintain consistent continuity of patient care and help to inform future decisions regarding patient management and MI examinations [23].

The professional NPs in a study by Makanjee et al. were eager to expand their scope of practice, specifically to include the interpretation of radiographs [24]. Based on their wish to provide feedback to patients who are anxious or in transition between MI and another point of contact and to compile evidence-based nursing notes. NPs are usually the first to prepare the patient for MI examinations, read the radiological interpretation report, and provide the interpretation to the clinician. Hence, it is very important for the NPs to have a basic understanding of Chest radiographic findings to sharpen their assessment skills, promote patient safety, and alter their actions to benefit the patient [25]. Several studies have shown evidence that NPs can interpret plain radiographic, CT, and ultrasound images through experiential learning or formal training [25, 26]. The evolving nature of this role has occurred in response to emergency departments' necessity to discover innovative ways to improve service delivery also linked to other subspecialties within the hospital is the timeliness of the accessibility and delivery of these images. A solution could be to device process metrics to provide an indication on aspects of the value of delivery in terms of the timeliness of the information delivery and its applicability to appropriate levels of specialization and subspecialties to interpret [5].

## 4. NP roles and responsibilities in the immediate MI environment

NPs caring for patients in MI started in the 1970s because of multimodality, cutting-edge imaging technologies. Thereby, the potential to improve efficiency, grow service lines, and improve the visibility of MI departments. A challenge in the immediate MI working environment could be adapting from having stable nursing care plans and routines to the frequency of changing plans when a patient is a switch between modalities. In close collaboration with multidisciplinary teams in imaging services, ensuring also that policies, guidelines, and protocols are complied with and contribute toward enhancing effective improvements [24, 27, 28]. For example, during the general or plain radiographic examination depending on the patient's characteristics, the competency of the radiographer and equipment ensuring the patient's comfort while in the MI examination room, the orienting and supporting the patient's immobility during the exam, interdependent on patient cooperation, such as holding breath for a while. Providing a calm and relaxed environment for the patient is indeed vital. Complexities may arise when patients require sedation, especially in the pediatric population group. Often requires scheduling in coordination with the hospital's specialized nursing care center and medical specialist. According to Ruess and the authors, there were inconsistencies in terms of the method of administration and type of medications. A confounding factor was the variable levels of experience [29]. To resolve this issue representatives from nursing staff and physicians from pediatric radiology, pediatric, anesthesia, and quality services representatives, formed a multidisciplinary team. The review entailed using institutional and national regulatory authorities' guidelines and protocols to standardize the ordering process, pre-sedation history and physical examination, physician training and staffing, and sedation medication protocols. Implementing a sedation pathway enhanced the safety, effectiveness, and efficiency of sedation medication for routine diagnostic imaging procedures [29].

Another area is the fluoroscopic imaging procedures where NPs play a chore role whether it be outside or within the immediate MI section. The Fluoroscopy MI technique uses ionizing radiation to obtain real-time moving and or static images of internal structures and functions on a display screen and guide the procedures [30]. NPs take on numerous roles during fluoroscopically guided interventions (FGI) procedures ranging from working in a radiation environment to operating fluoroscopy equipment where permissible by law. The patient care processes pre-, during post-fluoroscopic examinations. For instance, to improve the quality of the images and to obtain a safe report, before starting the exam, the nursing professional checks if the patient has prepared as requested when scheduling the exam. Fluoroscopic examinations like other modalities such as CT, MRI, and US include the administration of contrast agents associated with the patient's physiological condition. During this process, NPs together with MI professional team include safe medication management in contemporary clinical practice. Record keeping is central for risk management (e.g., contrast reactions and extravasations) and medico-legal reasons. Knowledgeable of the associated risk with contrast agent administrations include the knowledge of characteristics of the type of contrast agents and its suitability among other in conjunction with the catheter selection, cannulation site, etc. [7]. Occupational risks include radiation exposure, slips, trips, falls, and potential head injuries, along with potential exposure to chemotherapy, bodily fluids, and other pathogens, which are the most common risks faced by multidisciplinary team members including medical imaging NPs [31].

## 5. Nurse practitioner roles and responsibilities outside the immediate MI environment

Most hospitals are equipped with the provision of MI services away from the immediate MI section. In this section, the focus shifts toward, critical care units, theater, ward MI examinations, and remote mobile MI services [17]. As already mentioned, NPs are vital in the management of patients for ionizing and non-ionizing MI examinations. In the previous section, the role of non-medical imaging NPs was briefly touched upon in terms of handovers and the importance of an effective efficient manner of communication information exchange. An integral component is the competency, roles, and responsibilities of the contemporary multidisciplinary team members in aligning, coordinating, cooperating, collaborating, and communicating in critical decision-making processes and procedures regarding MI examinations protocols in maintaining and sustaining the seamless clinical medical CoC and wellbeing of the persons. For example, peripherally inserted central catheter insertion by NPs under fluoroscopy guidance has been shown to be a safe and suitable alternative to radiologist insertion with similar technical success and similar long-term complication rates. It could have flow-on effects in terms of cost reduction, provision of technical ward support, and allowing radiology medical staff the time to perform other fluoroscopic or angiographic procedures [32]. Central to and interwoven is technology as an enabler, facilitator, and mediating the network of interactional processes in achieving these seamless quality outcomes in patient management. The overarching and golden thread to be considered, is the holistic care and safety culture.

Pros could be ease of access where transferring a patient to the MI section could result in compromised care in terms of their unstable medical condition affecting both the treatment and nursing care. Also, requires careful consideration in terms of radiation safety and the quality of the completeness of an MI examination. For example, one needs to ensure that the physical environment is radiation safety compliant, like the thickness of the walls in theater and critical care units. Considerations include radiation protection control measures during mobile radiography such as bed distancing and protecting patients, themselves, and members of the public visiting the ward/unit. So, the timing of an MI examination, if possible, can be negotiated to avoid unnecessary exposure to the public unless critical. Some of the most common MI examinations performed is the chest radiographic imaging examinations. The most common indications for performing portable MI examinations are to check for positions of tracheostomies, nasogastric tubes (NGs), central lines or central venous catheters (CVCs), trauma injuries, pacemakers, and other medical conditions of patients who require special care. Other MI examinations can also be performed, but dependent on the type of MI equipment and its characteristics, the quality of radiographic images, and safety [17].

Prior to commencing a MI examination, a written MI request should be made. Apart from the medico-legal requirement and justification aspect, the radiographer needs to plan the imaging examination, select an appropriate image receptor, ensure the equipment is optimally functioning and appropriate imaging exposure parameters are selected and may require additional accessories such as immobilization aids. Assess the patient's condition in liaison with the NP. The NPs are responsible for the patient knowing condition and patient's needs. The radiographer and NP collaboratively coordinate the immobilizing, positioning of the patient, and the image receptor device to acquire the required radiographic projection of the body part of interest. At the end of the imaging examination, the NP or referring doctor should be informed of when the outcomes of the imaging examination are likely to be available [17].

## 6. An overview of shared roles and responsibilities on safety culture

An important aspect throughout any MI examination is aspects of infection control and cross-contamination. Any infection control measures should be communicated to the MI professionals and infection control protocols always be adhered to. Include the MI equipment and its accessories and radiation safety protective gear. For instance, theater and mobile MI equipment and its accessories should ideally be dedicated units kept on site. During an imaging examination, it is advisable to cover the image receptor with a suitable cover material (double-bagged if required) to prevent contamination from body fluids. Also, take into consideration that the material used will not create an artifact and is radiolucent. As would compromise the quality of the MI examination and risk the safety of the patient. When dealing with highly contagious infections wear appropriate personal protective equipment (PPE). All contaminated gear such as the covers and PPE placed in the correct waste bins. Occasionally, NP would be required to assist in the imaging of these patients. The principles of barrier nursing techniques of infection control are necessary. During this process, the role and responsibility of the radiographer and NPs knowledge of body part positioning, aligning of the image receptor, and following instructions from the radiographer is important in ensuring that safety is maintained without compromising the quality of the MI examination.

Following the MI radiation safety guidelines are significantly important. NPs should be knowledgeable about radiation safety rather than learning on the job from hearsay. Practical errors and feedback and annual training on radiation protection and safety and should be included in an occupational dose monitoring program. Basic radiation protection principles can be summarized as, time, distance, and shielding. All radiation protection strategies are fundamentally related to one or more of these rules. Using personal dosimeters ensures the management of the duration of stay in an area with high radiation levels and the monitoring of accumulated doses. Use radiation protective gear such as lead aprons, thyroid shields, and lead glasses. Justified by the role of the NP during fluoroscopic guided intervention who is in proximity monitoring the patient, an advocate for the patient, and reporting back all pertinent information related to potential safety concerns. A mobile lead shield that is transparent, at least on the upper half, can be used to create a protected area at the nurse workstation. NPs who take on the role of a procedure assistant will move around the room and therefore will require the same thickness apron in the front and back. Ceiling-suspended shields are also very effective at reducing radiation dose to the upper body and the lenses of the eyes [17, 33].

Like their MI professional counterparts, medical imaging NPs who are pregnant or planning to become pregnant do not need to modify their duties related to working in radiation environments [34]. Pregnant radiation workers should declare their pregnancy to a radiation safety officer and acquire a fetal dosimeter in addition to the occupational dosimeter worn under PRE at the level of the conceptus, used to monitor the dose to the conceptus. The dose to the conceptus is restricted to a much lower level than that of the worker [31].

## 7. Conclusions

In conclusion, this chapter provided a snapshot of the NPs integrated roles and responsibilities as part of the contemporary MI team both within and outside of an evolving technological medical imaging environment and service delivery. This chapter adds to the contribution, performance, and recognition of their work. Essentially, MI professionals (radiologists and radiographers) should acquaint themselves with the scope of practice of NPs and vice versa to achieve an optimal quality outcome for the patient. This could be achieved through sharing teaching, research, continuous professional development, evidence-based practice forums; working collaboratively in developing quality management improvement plans, protocols, and guidelines in the management of the patient. Lastly, at the regulatory professional level, the scope of the profession and practice to enhance the capabilities and standards of practice, and to provide Continuing Professional Development (CPD) to NP to keep up-to-date with any developments in the safety area.

## Conflict of interest

None.

## Author details

Chandra Rekha Makanjee
University of Canberra, Bruce, Australia

*Address all correspondence to: chandra.makanjee@canberra.edu.au

## References

[1] Park K. Health care of the community. In: Park K, editor. Park's Text Book of Preventive and Social Medicine. 20th ed. Jabalpur: Banarsidas Bhanot; 2009. pp. 780-800. DOI: 10.1007/978-981-19-6692-7_5

[2] Aggarwal A, Aeran H, Rathee M. Quality management in healthcare: The pivotal desideratum. Journal of Oral Biology and Craniofacial Research. 2019;**9**(2):180-182. DOI: 10.1016/j.jobcr.2018.06.006

[3] Ljungholm L, Edin-Liljegren A, Ekstedt M, Klinga C. What is needed for continuity of care and how can we achieve it?—Perceptions among multiprofessionals on the chronic care trajectory. BMC Health Services Research. 2022;**22**(1):1-5. DOI: 10.1186/s12913-022-08023-0

[4] Frija G, Blažić I, Frush DP, Hierath M, Kawooya M, Donoso-Bach L, et al. How to improve access to medical imaging in low-and middle-income countries? EClinicalMedicine. 2021;**38**:101034. DOI: 10.1016/j.eclinm.2021.101034

[5] Brady AP, Bello JA, Derchi LE, Fuchsjäger M, Goergen S, Krestin GP, et al. Radiology in the era of value-based healthcare: A multi-society expert statement from the ACR, CAR, ESR, IS3R, RANZCR, and RSNA. Canadian Association of Radiologists Journal. 2021;**72**(2):208-214. DOI: 10.1177/0846537120982567

[6] Hricak H, Abdel-Wahab M, Atun R, Mikhail Lette M, Paez D, Brink J, et al. Medical imaging and nuclear medicine: A lancet oncology commission. Lancet Oncology. 2021;**22**(4):e136-e172. DOI: 10.1016/S1470-2045(20):30751-8

[7] Acauan LV, Seda JM, Silva SCSB, Paes GO, Trotte LAC, Stipp MAC. The performance of the nursing team in outpatient radiology and diagnostic imaging services. Revista gaucha de enfermagem. 2022;**43**:e20210079. DOI: 0.1590/1983-1447.2022.20210079.en

[8] Lancet T. 2020: Unleashing the full potential of nursing. Lancet (London, England). 2019;**394**(10212):1879. DOI: 10.1016/s0140-6736(19)32794-1

[9] Birks M, Davis J, Smithson J, Cant R. Registered nurse scope of practice in Australia: An integrative review of the literature. Contemporary Nurse. 2016;**52**(5):522-543. DOI: 10.1080/10376178.2016.1238773

[10] Leslie K, Moore J, Robertson C, et al. Regulating health professional scopes of practice: Comparing institutional arrangements and approaches in the US, Canada, Australia and the UK. Human Resources for Health. 2021;**19**:15. DOI: 10.1186/s12960-020-00550-3

[11] Gleason K, Harkless G, Stanley J, Olson AP, Graber ML. The critical need for nursing education to address the diagnostic process. Nursing Outlook. 2021;**69**(3):362-369. DOI: 10.1016/j.outlook.2020.12.005

[12] Cantiello J, Kitsantas P, Moncada S, Abdul S. The evolution of quality improvement in healthcare: Patient-centered care and health information technology applications. Journal of Hospital Administration. 2016;**5**(2):62-68. DOI: 10.5430/jha.v5n2p62 4

[13] Carley A, Melrose S, Rempel G, Diehl-Jones W, Schwarz BA. Professional development needs of non-radiology nurses: An exploration of nurses' experiences caring for interventional

radiology patients. Journal of Radiology Nursing. 2021;**40**(2):146-151. DOI: 10.1016/j.jradnu.2020.12.011

[14] Proposed Legislative Changes to Authorise Core and Supplemental Clinical Activities Performed by Nurse Practitioners. Available from: https://www.health.act.gov.au/sites/default/files/2021-12/Consultation%20Paper_Final.pdf

[15] Ghanes K, Jouini O, Wargon M, Jemai Z. Modeling and analysis of triage nurse ordering in emergency departments. In: 2015 International Conference on Industrial Engineering and Systems Management (IESM). Seville, Spain: IEEE; 2015. pp. 228-235. DOI: 10.1109/IESM.2015.7380163

[16] Hughes DR, Jiang M, Duszak R. A comparison of diagnostic imaging ordering patterns between advanced practice clinicians and primary care physicians following office-based evaluation and management visits. JAMA Internal Medicine. 2015;**175**(1):101-107. DOI: 10.1001/jamainternmed.2014.6349

[17] Bwanga O. What nurses need to know about mobile radiography. British Journal of Nursing. 2020;**29**(18):1064-1067. DOI: 10.12968/bjon.2020.29.18.1064

[18] Solheim J, Storm R, Whitney J. Radiological imaging and the emergency department: Teamed for success. A patient-centered approach to emergent imaging practices. Journal of Radiology Nursing. 2018;**37**(2):69-72. DOI: 10.1016/j.jradnu

[19] Li Q, Yuan Y, Song G, Liu Y. Nursing analysis based on medical imaging technology before and after coronary angiography in cardiovascular medicine. Applied Bionics and Biomechanics. 2022;**2022**:3279068. DOI: 10.1155/2022/3279068. PMID: 35465185; PMCID: PMC9033406

[20] Ranschaert ER. The impact of information technology on radiology services: An overview. Journal of the Belgian Society of Radiology. 2016;**100**(1):93, 1-6. DOI: 10.5334/jbr-btr.1184

[21] Zadvinskis IM, Smith JG, Yen PY. Nurses' experience with health information technology: Longitudinal qualitative study. JMIR Medical Informatics. 2018;**6**(2):e8734. DOI: 10.2196/medinform.8734

[22] Abuzaid MM, Elshami W, Fadden SM. Integration of artificial intelligence into nursing practice. Health Technol (Berl). 2022;**12**(6):1109-1115. DOI: 10.1007/s12553-022-00697-0. Epub 2022 Sep 14. PMID: 36117522; PMCID: PMC9470236

[23] Walton ER, Gandhi S. Record keeping in radiology: Are we doing enough? The British Journal of Radiology. 2016;**89**(1068):20160586. DOI: 10.1259/bjr.20160586

[24] Makanjee CR, Bergh AM, Hoffmann WA. "So you are running between"—A qualitative study of nurses' involvement with diagnostic imaging in South Africa. Journal of Radiology Nursing. 2014;**33**(3):105-115. DOI: 10.1016/j.jradnu.2013.12.005

[25] Singh J, Sharma T. Unveiling the basics of chest radiography for nurses. Journal of Primary Care Specialties. 2022;**3**(3):45. DOI: 10.4103/jopcs.jopcs_9_22

[26] Swamy V, Brainin P, Biering-Sørensen T, Platz E. Ability of non-physicians to perform and interpret lung ultrasound: A systematic review. European Journal of Cardiovascular Nursing. 2019;**18**(6):474-483. DOI: 10.1177/1474515119845972

[27] Murphy A, Ekpo E, Steffens T, Neep MJ. Radiographic image interpretation by Australian radiographers: A systematic review. Journal of Medical Radiation Sciences. 2019;**66**(4):269-283. DOI: 10.1002/jmrs.356

[28] Schlunegger MC, Aeschlimann S, Palm R, Zumstein-Shaha M. Competencies and scope of practice of nurse practitioners in primary health care: A scoping review protocol. JBI Evidence Synthesis. 2021;**19**(4):899-905. DOI: 10.11124/JBIES-20-00554

[29] Ruess L, O'Connor SC, Mikita CP, Creamer KM. Sedation for pediatric diagnostic imaging: Use of pediatric and nursing resources as an alternative to a radiology department sedation team. Pediatric Radiology. 2002;**32**(7):505-510. DOI: 10.1007 /s00247-002-0712-9

[30] Hunter T, Jayasekera N, Roach R. Safer mobile fluoroscopy in the trauma theatre: A survey of orthopaedic registrars and theatre staff. The Bulletin of the Royal College of Surgeons of England. 2014;**96**(6):206-208. DOI: 10.1308/rcsbull.2014.96.6.206

[31] Jones AK, Ramirez JA III. The role of the radiology nurse in managing radiation dose during fluoroscopically guided interventional procedures. Journal of Radiology Nursing. 2022;**41**(3):201-206. DOI: 10.1016/j.jradnu.2022.05.006

[32] Askey J, Clements W. A single-center experience of fluoroscopic-guided peripherally inserted central catheter insertion by nursing staff: Rationale and clinical outcomes. Journal of Radiology Nursing. 2019;**38**(3):155-157. DOI: 10.1016/j.jradnu.2019.06.004

[33] Chida K. What are useful methods to reduce occupational radiation exposure among radiological medical workers, especially for interventional radiology personnel? Radiological Physics and Technology. 2022;**15**(2):101-115. DOI: 10.1007/s12194-022-00660-8

[34] Dauer LT, Miller DL, Schueler B, Silberzweig J, Balter S, Bartal G, et al. Occupational radiation protection of pregnant or potentially pregnant workers in IR: A joint guideline of the Society of Interventional Radiology and the cardiovascular and interventional radiological Society of Europe. Journal of Vascular and Interventional Radiology. 2015;**26**(2):171-181. DOI: 10.1016/j.jvir.2014.11.026

Chapter 6

# Palliative Care

*Marvin J. Gordon*

## Abstract

Palliative care bridges the gap between medically focused care with case management support, and hospice with focus on comfort only in the last 6 months of life. A multidisciplinary palliative team provides support, both medical and psycho-social, regardless of time to end of life. Patients do not forego any treatments or interrupt any current physician relationships when enrolling in palliative care. Programs may be in-patient, clinic based, home based, telehealth or a combination of venues. 24-hour availability is encouraged. Coordination with the existing medical team and the health plan is a key to success. Periodic rounding between the palliative providers and the health plan team facilitates making the managed care system seamless for members and providers. The most common adult diagnosis is cancer, but severe progressive disease of any organ system may be appropriate for referral. Some patients may stabilize or even improve. Pediatric palliative care is somewhat different with the diagnosis more likely being genetic, developmental, or neurologic. Severe diseases in children may be chronic and end of life discussions difficult. Communication skills facilitate advance care planning discussions whether advance directive or POLST. Palliative care is a cost-effective program that improves patient care without the patient relinquishing existing benefits.

**Keywords:** palliative care, hospice, advance care planning, severe progressive disease, patient support

## 1. Introduction

Palliative care is a relatively new field that has expanded over the past 15 years. Palliative care uses a specially trained team to support patients with severe progressive disease and their caregivers. The World Health Organization describes palliative care as "… improves the quality of life of patients and that of their families who are facing challenges associated with life-threatening illness, whether physical, psychological, social, or spiritual" [1]. This includes addressing practical needs and providing bereavement counseling. It offers a support system to help patients live as actively as possible until death.

Palliative care is indicated for a wide range of severe progressive diseases. The most common diseases needing adult palliative care include cardiovascular diseases (38.5%), cancer (34%), chronic respiratory diseases (10.3%), AIDS (5.7%) and diabetes (4.6%) [1]. Other conditions include kidney failure, chronic liver disease, autoimmune diseases, neurological disease, dementia, and congenital anomalies.



IntechOpen

Symptoms encountered during palliative care most commonly include pain and difficulty in breathing. Opioids are essential for managing pain and other symptoms. Palliative care is about the quality of living, recognizing that dying is a normal process, and palliative care does not hasten nor postpone death.

A landmark randomized controlled study of patients with metastatic non-small-cell lung cancer demonstrated that the addition of early palliative care, as compared to standard oncologic care alone, not only resulted in less depression, improved quality of life, fewer hospitalizations and emergency department visits, and less aggressive interventions, but the palliative group lived significantly longer [2]. Although this is not meant to imply that palliative care will always prolong life, it does suggest that palliative care certainly does not hasten death.

Palliative care integrates the psychological and spiritual aspects of patient care and offers a support system for the family, the caregivers, and the patients. The patient does not "give up" access to existing providers or any existing benefits including therapies intended to prolong life, such as chemotherapy or radiation therapy, and other disease focused investigations or therapies as well as treating any clinical complications. Palliative care is based on the needs of the patient, not on the patient's prognosis. It is appropriate at any age and at any stage in a serious illness, and it can be provided along with curative treatment.

## 2. Defining palliative care versus hospice versus case management versus community care coordination with community health workers (CHW)

For **Palliative Care**, the patient retains all of their disease focused benefits, adding support in addition to disease focused treatments. Palliative care does not require a prognosis shorter than 6 months. Hospice is a program in which the member foregoes curative focused treatment and focuses on comfort only for the hospice diagnosis.

**Hospice Care** is defined by Medicare as being for the terminally ill (with a life expectancy of 6 months or less) for members having Medicare Part A (Hospital Insurance), for which you accept comfort care (palliative care) instead of care to cure your illness.

Medicare-certified hospice care is usually given in the home or other facility where they live, like a nursing home. Patients can also get hospice care in an inpatient hospice facility if needed. "Original Medicare" will still pay for covered benefits for any health problems that are not part of your terminal illness and related conditions. Once the patient chooses hospice care, the hospice benefit will usually cover everything needed.

Specific for patient's illness, the hospice team will create a plan of care that can include any or all these services:

- Doctors' services.
- Nursing and medical services.
- Durable medical equipment for pain relief and symptom management.
- Medical supplies, like bandages or catheters.
- Drugs for pain management.

*DOI: http://dx.doi.org/10.5772/intechopen.109390*

- Aide and homemaker services.
- Physical therapy services.
- Occupational therapy services.
- Speech-language pathology services.
- Social services.
- Dietary counseling.
- Spiritual and grief counseling for patient and the family.
- Short-term inpatient care for pain and symptom management. This care must be in a Medicare-approved facility, like a hospice facility, hospital, or skilled nursing facility that contracts with the hospice.
- Inpatient care
- Respite care (which is care received in a Medicare-approved facility like an inpatient facility, hospital, or nursing home), so that the usual caregiver (like a family member or friend) can rest. The hospice provider will arrange this for the patient. Respite care givers can stay up to 5 days each time respite care is required. Respite care can be provided more than once, but only on an occasional basis.
- Any other services Medicare covers to manage pain and other symptoms related to the terminal illness and related conditions, as the hospice team recommends.

Initial certification is done by the patient's usual doctor or the hospice doctor. After 6 months, hospice care can be continued provided that the hospice medical director or hospice doctor recertifies (at a face-to-face meeting) that the patient is still terminally ill.

As a hospice patient, the patient always has the right to stop hospice care at any time.

Medicare will not cover any of these once the hospice benefit starts:

- Treatment intended to cure the terminal illness and/or related conditions.
- Prescription drugs to cure the hospice illness (rather than for symptom control or pain relief).
- Care from any hospice provider that wasn't set up by the hospice medical team. However, the patient can still see his/her regular doctor or nurse practitioner if that provider has been chosen to be the attending medical professional who helps supervise the hospice care.
- Room and board. Medicare does not cover room and board for hospice care in your home or if you live in a nursing home or a hospice inpatient facility.

**Hospital outpatient care (like in an emergency room), hospital inpatient care, or ambulance transportation** must be arranged by your hospice provider unless it is unrelated to your hospice diagnosis.

**Case Management** is process of assessment, evaluation, care coordination, education, and advocacy to meet an individual's and family's comprehensive health needs. This includes continuity and transition while promoting quality and cost-effective outcomes. Clinical as well as psycho-social issues are addressed. Several types of case management exist:

- Managing patients with high-cost medical conditions. The goal is to coordinate the care to both improve continuity and quality of care while lowering costs.
- Chronic care which may be disease specific
- Catastrophic or large claim management programs
- Maternity case management programs
- Transitional management programs including in-patient discharge planning

The case management team may include

- Nurses
- Physicians
- Social workers
- Pharmacists
- Behavioral health specialists
- Care givers
- Community resources

Another growing trend is the use of **Community Health Workers** (CHW), non-licensed trusted members of the community, to navigate and assist patients in obtaining community services to address social determinants of health (SDoH) and coordinate with traditional health care. Typical SDoH would include:

- Homelessness/shelter
- Food security
- Safety
- Transportation
- Financial

- Education
- Post incarceration
- Behavioral health
- Adverse childhood experiences

CHW programs are for any patient in need of navigation and support regardless of prognosis or severity of illness. CHWs do not manage symptoms since they are not licensed to provide medical care. Some CHWs may be specially trained to handle advance care planning.

**Figure 1** compares case management, palliative care, and hospice.

- Case management: the primary focus is disease focused led by the usual physician driven health care team. Case Manager (CM) and Social Worker (SW) staff assist as needed especially addressing psycho-social needs and coordination of care. These members tend to have catastrophic or chronic illness but are not necessarily nearing the end of life. Although advance directives are encouraged, they are not critical. The patient continues with their existing medical team and retains all existing benefits including disease focused and/or curative treatment.

- Palliative care: although palliative is appropriate at any stage of illness, these patients are usually within their last 1–2 years of life. In addition to their existing health care team, an additional team of physicians, nurses, social workers, and coordinators is added. These patients usually have severe progressive disease. Advance care planning (ACP) is extremely important, and the patient and family should be engaged in this discussion, hopefully with documentation and

| CASE MANAGEMENT | PALLIATIVE CARE | HOSPICE BENEFITS |
|---|---|---|
| Chronic / complex disease- not contemplating death | End of life 1-2 years and/or chronic / complex disease | End of life 6 months |
| Concurrent with curative care | Symptom relief concurrent with curative | Symptom relief only<br>NO curative (for terminal illness) |
| Primary care physician (PCP) and specialist | PCP, specialist, and palliative consultant | Hospice team including physician |
| Complex Case Management (CCM) RN/social worker (SW) | Integrated team approach MD/NP/RN/SW | Integrated team plus aides, chaplain, and respite benefit |
| Focus: Curative treatment by usual medical team with support for psycho-social issues | Focus: Transition from curative only to symptom management and goals of care | Focus: Symptom relief by the hospice team with NO curative treatment of the terminal illness |
| Advance directive<br>+/- Physician Orders for Life-Sustaining Treatment (POLST) | Advance directive<br>POLST discussion | Advance directive and signed POLST |

**Figure 1.**
*Comparison of case management to palliative care to hospice.*

distribution of ACP documents. Coordination between the palliative team and the usual medical team is an imperative. The patient is receiving both disease-focused/curative treatment and intensive supportive treatment.

- Hospice: is specifically for those with a prognosis of 6 months or less, although renewals of the 6-month period are possible. The patient is focused on comfort care only for the terminal diagnosis. There is no curative treatment being given. Illness not related to the terminal diagnosis is still treated. Advance care planning with documentation is essential since limiting futile medical care at the end of life is a goal. The hospice team will direct the care of the member unless the patient designates his/her PCP to perform that function. Hospice may be revoked at any time.

- Community Health Workers: are trusted sources of navigators from the local community who are not medically licensed but can assist in addressing social determinants of health (SD0H) needs regardless of the health status. Some CHWs have training in advance care planning discussions. CHWs can be part of the palliative care team.

## 3. Referral criteria

The most common referral criteria for adult palliative care include

- Severe progressive disease although severe progressive disease can be stabilized or even cured

- Death not unexpected in 1–2 years although predicting the timetable for death may not always be accurate

- Symptoms uncontrolled with the most common symptoms being pain, weakness, shortness of breath, nausea, and depression

- Support needed which includes psycho-social support as well as medical

- Advance care planning (ACP) needed with an advance directive (AD) advisable for everyone and the POLST (Provider Orders for Life Sustaining Treatment) for those nearing end of life (EOL)

## 4. Models

The most common models used to deliver palliative care include

- Hospital based: A palliative team is available to consult with in-patients and emergency room patients. They may have an out-patient clinic for follow up or they may need to refer to an out-patient program

- Clinic based: the palliative team is able to see the patient in an out-patient clinic.

- Home based; the palliative team is able to see the patient in the home.

- Telehealth: the home visits are virtual using audio-video or audio only. A hybrid model can be used in which the nurse or community health care worker does the home visit and oversees a telehealth visit with a physician, nurse, or social worker.

## 5. Sources of referrals

Most referrals are made by in-patient case managers, discharge planners, health plan case managers, concurrent review nurses, transition care management nurses, or hospitalists. Other common sources of referrals include primary care physicians, specialty care physicians such as oncologists and nephrologists, or out-patient clinic staff. Although emergency rooms see many palliative candidates, referrals from the ED (emergency department) are less frequent unless special support staff are available to the emergency room for consultation. Data mining looking for high cost and high-risk members through claims data is limited since there is a significant lag time between claims data being processed and the actual sentinel events that indicate the need for palliative support.

Data mining for high-risk members usually requires risk stratification programs such as I Pro (Impact Pro®). A population is stratified from the sickest of the sick down to healthy members. Data mining looks at claims including cost, pharmacy, inpatient utilization, ED utilization, age, sex, diagnosis, demographics, and even social determinants of health. Another tool is the Charlson Co-morbidity Index which looks at multiple co-morbidities to create a score. In any case, prognostication is difficult. Even though these tools may stratify, there is no guarantee that the prediction for any single patient will be correct. Prognosticating the timetable for end of life is even more difficult. Although studies do show the efficacy of palliative care in the last several months of life, predicting when that end-of-life period begins is not always accurate.

The types of patients referred to palliative care may vary and include end-of-life, chronic illness, catastrophic illness, and/or being inpatient. Social determinants of health may also require significant attention. Different illnesses may have different patterns of functional decline (**Figure 2**). Cancer members may remain quite

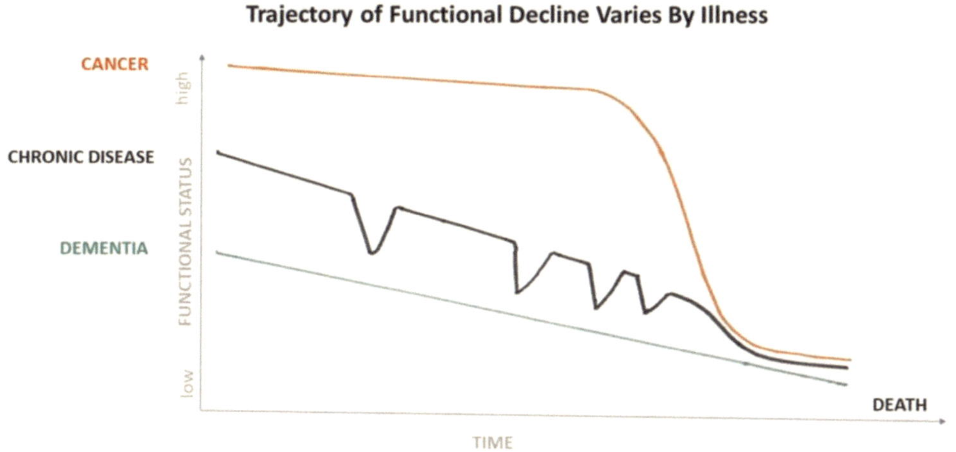


**Figure 2.**
*Trajectory of functional decline variation by type illness.*

functional despite significant disease. When the functional decline begins, the rate of decline may be fairly rapid, not allowing much time for interventions at end of life. Chronic diseases such as heart failure may have a slower decline with episodic acute exacerbations. Although they may recover from the exacerbation, they are not recovering back to their previous state of health. The decline is often not noticed since the focus is on the miraculous improvement from of the exacerbation. The exacerbations may increase in frequency and have a slower recovery until the final exacerbation occurs, from which the patient does not recover. The third type of functional decline is exemplified by dementia. In the absence of an acute complication, the course is a slow steady decline which may last for years. These varying scenarios make prognostication difficult.

An interesting tool for prognostication is the "surprise question". Rather than asking how long a patient is expected to live, the question is "would you be surprised if this patient died within the next 1-2 years?" The efficacy of this tool is debatable and does vary by disease category.

## 6. Pediatric palliative care

Pediatric palliative care is different than adult palliative in many ways.

- Treating a whole family, including siblings
- Pediatric diagnoses are different (genetic, development, metabolic, neurologic)
- High claims data mining does not always identify candidates (sick neonates are usually the highest cost group)
- Many times, it is catastrophic issues (trauma, burns, complications of appendicitis) that are high-cost severe illnesses in children
- Medicaid high-cost pediatric chronic disease is often carved out to special sick children programs such as CCS (California Children's Services) in California
- Candidates may be better identified by ICD-10 codes than high cost
- Pediatric diagnoses are often more chronic
- Prognosis determination is difficult in children
- Children have limited skills for verbal expression
- Expressive therapies such as art therapy, music therapy, and play therapy may be used
- Massage therapy can be used for symptom relief
- Hospice and DNR (Do Not Resuscitate) are emotionally difficult decisions in children

Identifying children for referral to palliative care is difficult since they often have disease that is chronic but may have exacerbations for which palliative care is appropriate. The California Department of Health Care Services did define criteria for pediatric palliative for Medicaid members [3]. The criteria were:

- "There is documentation of a life-threatening diagnosis which can include but is not limited to … ."
    - "Conditions for which curative treatment is possible"
    - "Conditions requiring intensive long-term treatment"
    - "Progressive conditions for which treatment is exclusively palliative"
    - "Conditions involving severe non-progressive disability"
- "The member may continue to access both palliative care and curative care until the condition improves, stabilizes, or results in death."
- "MCPs [Managed Care Plan] may discontinue palliative care that is no longer medically necessary or no longer reasonable"

## 7. Structure

The palliative team personnel can vary. Some programs emphasize the physician and nurse practitioner. This is very important in cases in which control of symptoms and disease management are a major factor. In some cases where there is a behavioral health concern or social determinants of health play a major role, the social worker may play the key role. Looking at both health care and social issues, the nurse, either licensed vocational or registered nurse may play the key role. Often the patient will express a preference for nurse or social worker visits rather than physicians and nurse practitioners. For telehealth, having a community health worker may be helpful to assist the patient in setting up a telehealth video visit in the home with the physician or nurse. The approach to staffing may vary depending on other lines of business that the vendor performs. Those vendors who also do hospice may have more physician involvement. Organizations who do home health, may be more nurse centered.

The frequency of visits can be flexible since not every member has the same needs. A "typical" frequency of home visits may be 1 physician/NP visit every 1–2 months, a nurse every week, a social worker once a month, and coordinators and spiritual advisors as needed. These services are supplemented with phone communication. Obviously, not every week would be the same with more visits some weeks and less visits some weeks. If monthly case rates (fixed fee per month) are used, the rate can be adjusted for different levels of care. Those averaging the predetermined number of visits specified in the contract may get paid the full fixed fee per month; but if the average number of visits decreases, the case rate payment can be decreased proportionally. Case rates can also allow fee for service visits above and beyond the case rate services if exceptional services are required. The palliative provider can also work under a fee for service contract. However, the fee for service contract may require more prior authorization or documentation. Case rates can also be adjusted if the member only was enrolled for part of the month. For in-patient and clinic visits, palliative services are often billed as hospital consults or office visits respectively.

The actual provider of the palliative care, the vendor, has several different models. The payer can contract directly with local vendors. This has the advantage of using vendors known in the community. Depending on the size of the service area, home visits may be relatively easy. Larger national companies can be contracted, but then that company needs to either contract with local vendors or set up a network of employed providers if face to face visits are needed. The use of telehealth with or without community health worker making home visits does allow the palliative provider to cover a much larger service area.

## 8. Outcomes and disposition

Overall, studies have shown that there is very high satisfaction with home based palliative care programs [4]. In general, utilization of the hospital and emergency department (ED) decrease, overall health care cost decreases (mostly due to in-patient and ED savings), savings are greater when the patient is closer to end of life, and certain diagnoses like cancer are more likely show savings than chronic illness like dementia [5]. Cost reduction does vary by insurance product with largest savings seen in the commercial product, probably because the unit cost is highest compared to Medicare and Medicaid.

Some patients referred to palliative care will choose hospice instead once they understand their options. Of patients qualifying for palliative care, about 15–20% of members will refuse the program. Reasons for refusal include misunderstanding despite explanations, fear that they will receive less care, cultural beliefs, fear of talking about death, family disagreement, or wanting privacy without anyone in their home. Physicians may not make the referral due to a misunderstanding that existing benefits continue, fear that they are giving up, not wanting to discourage the member, or not having the time for a series of end-of-life discussions. Often the physician does not understand the referral process or even the availability of the program.

Patients referred to palliative care may subsequently transfer to hospice, die, move out of the area, change insurance coverage, refuse services after enrollment, or actually improve such that they do not need further palliative care.

## 9. Advance directives

Advance Care Planning (ACP) is a process of discussing and then documenting a patient's wishes for health care. If the patient becomes incapable of making his/her health care decisions, then two questions arise. First, who can make those decisions for the patient (i.e. who is the patient's legal agent), and second, are the patients preferences known (and preferably documented)? Part of the discussion is an education of the patient and any family or significant others who the patient may want to be included in this process. The goal is to make informed decisions and then document before a catastrophic event occurs that leaves the patient unable to make their own decisions. Without written preferences, family members may disagree as to what the patient would really want. The patient and family may not understand all of the options. For example, a DNR (do not resuscitate) order may mean do nothing if the heart stops, or do only electrical stimulation, or administer drugs but no chest

*DOI: http://dx.doi.org/10.5772/intechopen.109390*

compressions. The patient may want CPR (cardio-pulmonary resuscitation) but would not want to remain on a ventilator (breathing machine) if there is no hope of recovery. Decisions could also include feeding tubes, dialysis (artificial kidney), surgery, hospitalization, or certain other treatments. The patient may refuse a certain treatment or agree to a limited trial of a treatment to be discontinued if recovery is not expected. If the directions are not clear, the designated agent would have the authority to intervene and make decisions.

ACP documents fall into two categories. The advance directive (AD) asks the patient to name the person, the agent, who would make medical decisions on their behalf should the patient be unable to do so. This gives the agent Durable Power of Attorney for Health Care. An alternate agent may also be named should the first choice not be available. The AD would also contain a general statement whether the patient's preference is to do anything possible to prolong life, or to limit interventions if there is no hope of recovery or regaining consciousness. A second question is whether the patient wants relief from pain even if it may hasten death. Other requests may be made such as type of burial or religious preferences. The AD can be notarized or signed by two witnesses who are not the agent.

The second document is the POLST (Provider Order for Life Sustaining Treatment). If the state does not allow nurse practitioners or physicians assistants to sign this order, the POLST is referenced as a Physician Order for Life Sustaining Treatment. Some states call this a MOLST (Medical Order for Life Sustaining Treatment). The POLST or MOLST is a specific order signed by the patient or his/her agent, and a physician or nurse practitioner (NP) or physician's assistant (PA) if allowed. The exact form may vary by state, but the content is similar. Does the patient want to be resuscitated? Does the patient not want to be on a ventilator (breathing machine) at all, or only for a limited period? Does the patient not want a feeding tube at all, or just for a limited period? The form also addresses wishes for hospitalization, intravenous fluids, or antibiotics. The POLST or MOLST must be signed by the patient (or his/her agent) and the physician (or NP or PA if allowed).

ACP discussions may require a series of meetings, since there is a lot of education, and the decision making may not be simple. Even if documents are created, periodic review is helpful since the patient's clinical status may change or multiple parties involved may forget what was said. The ACP documents can be revoked or amended at any time. If documents are generated and signed, it is important to distribute the documents to the appropriate parties like the patient, the agent, other participating family members, primary care physician, specialist physicians, and hospitals. For cases closer to the end of life (EOL), a copy of the advance directive may be placed on the refrigerator door in the home so the paramedics would have access to it. Some states have created a registry where the advance directives can be stored for easy access by medical personnel.

The logistics of ACP conversations can very. The primary care physician or specialist may have the conversation. However, the physician must be willing to devote time to this process including follow up meetings, be familiar with the process, and be willing to initiate what may be perceived as an uncomfortable subject. In the hospital, case managers or social workers may work with the patient and family, but usually when end of life or limiting interventions is the current issue. There are companies who specialize in doing advance directives. Usually, they take a telehealth approach. However, the personnel making the calls may vary between being a physician, a nurse, or a behavioral health trained person. Some community health workers are trained on doing advance directives.

## 10. Rounding

Communication concerning palliative care patients is critical because most of these patients are quite complex. On the other hand, not everything about a palliative patient can necessarily be addressed at one sitting since there are so many aspects to palliative care that can be discussed. Therefore, the communication or "rounding" has two aspects. One is the structure of the presentation, and the other is the content of the conversation.

The structure of the communication follows the SBAR format. This is a communication method developed in the airline industry to improve communication between pilots and co-pilots to avoid airplane accidents. The technique should shorten the conversation by "getting to the point". The acronym is:

- **S** is "situation": a brief description of why we are having this conversation, usually because there is some "problem" we wish to discuss

- **B** is "background": a brief capsule summary of the historical events that have lead up to this conversation

- **A** is "assessment": what are the current facts that the caller or presenter has found that should help us solve the problem.

- **R** is "recommendation": why is the caller calling and what is their recommendation as to what to do

In the medical world, this may be the typical emergency phone call at 3: 00 AM from the nurse to the doctor on call. If the conversation goes on for more that 3–5 minutes, the doctor usually interrupts with "why are you calling and what do you want me to do?" This suggests that the nurse is giving too much detail on the background and is not getting to the assessment and recommendation.

An example of SBAR in the world of palliative members for non-emergent presentation (such as nurse to medical director), would be:

S: I have a 63 year old male with hepatocellular cancer complicated by portal vein thrombosis and end stage liver disease with a prognosis 3–6- months.

B: The patient's course has been complicated by pain, altered mental status due to liver disease, portal vein thrombosis, endocarditis, and a stroke. Lactulose is being titrated for encephalopathy. Morphine is being given for pain. Trans-arterial radio embolization has been used in the past for pain remediation. Patient is on anticoagulation.

A: The patient agrees to a DNR but is not ready for hospice. His vision is failing due to cataracts and he really wants to see the Superbowl. Pain is not well controlled on morphine. Lactulose is effective and diarrhea is minimal. He has a supportive family and wants to be with them as much as possible.

R: We need to evaluate the pain … repeat radio-embolization is a consideration. The patient states it worked before. The patient wants cataract surgery. We should evaluate him for that. We need a signed POLST for the DNR. Continue the lactulose, morphine, and anticoagulants.

That is a very complicated patient presented in a relatively short-focused format. This allows plenty of time for the physician and nurse to further discuss the nurse recommendations and see if the medical director has any additional recommendations.

Looking at the content presented, the information falls into five categories.

- Medical:
    - Diagnosis
    - Prognosis
    - Symptoms
    - Medications and treatments
    - Current medical team
    - Hospitalizations and ED visits
- Functional status
    - Level
    - Trend
- Support system
    - Family
    - Caregivers
    - Spiritual
- SDoH (Social Determinants of Health)
    - Housing
    - Financial
    - Food security
    - Transportation
    - Safety
    - Behavioral health
- Advance Care Panning (ACP)
    - Advance directive
    - POLST
    - Series of discussions

The key to the conversations with the patient and family is not being judgmental, listening, asking open ended questions, showing empathy, and building a trusting relationship. The patient does have a right to determine how much they want to know, when they want to make their decisions, and what those decisions are.

## 11. Many faces of palliative care

Case Study 1: 63-year-old with hepatocellular cancer complicated by portal vein thrombosis and end stage liver disease. His prognosis was 3–6- months. The course was further complicated by endocarditis and a stroke. The patient's goal was to see the Super Bowl and he was not ready for hospice. He did agree to a Do Not Resuscitate (DNR) order. He did undergo cataract surgery. Lactulose was adjusted to control hepatic encephalopathy. Due to increasing pain the patient underwent trans-arterial radioembolization (radioactive microspheres injected into the hepatic artery) with improvement. Over 2 years he had 2 emergency admissions and 2 elective admits. Despite his poor prognosis, he survived for 2 years. He did convert to hospice 2 days before his death at home. He did get to see 2 Super Bowls.

This case exemplifies a patient with end stage cancer requiring both supportive and medical care such that he outlived his prognosis and enjoyed a high quality of life despite his diagnosis.

Case Study 2: 54-year-old with an Intracerebral bleed, currently on tracheotomy, ventilator, ventriculoperitoneal (V-P) shunt, and gastrostomy tube (G tube). She is in a long-term care subacute facility and had several acute-stay admits over the past year. She is scheduled for an elective admit for decubitus ulcer surgery. She never regained consciousness during 30-day acute hospitalization. She is full code, divorced with two daughters, ages 18 and 22, and has two siblings out of state. The case was presented to the palliative medical director at rounds, discussed with the subacute attending and case manager, the goals of care were reviewed, and POLST (Provider Orders for Life Sustaining Treatment) discussions were started with family.

The issue was raised why member is full code and whether family is aware that member will not wake up. The family was not aware that member will not wake up. The family expresses the wish to not keep mother alive "like this" recognizing the that decubitus ulcers can be painful.

The subacute attending concurred with decision to discontinue the ventilator. Palliative care arranges to discontinue vent with a palliative case manager, social worker, and spiritual advisor present. Time was allowed for the out of state relatives to join the daughters to be present when the ventilator was discontinued.

This is a case of palliative care addressing end of life wishes, advance care planning, and avoiding futile medical care.

Case Study 3: A 45-year-old presented with multiple emergency visits and admissions for abdominal wall infection. Five months prior, the member had undergone an abdominal hernia repair with placement of a mesh into the abdominal wall. The patient is having ED or acute admits 1–2 times per month. The member has abdominal pain and infection of an open wound at the hernia repair site. Oxycodone has been prescribed fairly regularly along with frequent antibiotics.

The member has filled all prescriptions for antibiotics and kept follow-up appointments with her surgeon and PCP. The surgeon was consulted as to why the mesh, the foreign material in the wound, has not been removed. The surgeon agrees that removal of the mesh is indicated, but he feels the surgery is too difficult for him to do due to obesity and scar tissue. The palliative team contacted a university-associated bariatric surgeon who agreed to do surgery, which was successful, and the wound healed. The course has been complicated by clostridium difficile, recurrent diarrhea, intermittent nausea and vomiting, and depression but with only occasional emergency department visits or admits.

This case seems to be a patient with severe progressive disease, but it is curable disease if the medical condition is treated properly. In this case the key intervention by the palliative team was to make the appropriate specialist referral.

Case Study 4: 65 year old, homeless patient with severe COPD requiring intermittent oxygen, continues smoking, and with multiple visits to the ED and hospital is referred to palliative care.

He had lost his job as a caretaker about 6 months prior. He now lives in his Lincoln Navigator SUV and he likes living there. He has portable oxygen and still smokes. He goes to senior centers for warmth, food, and socialization. He keeps some PCP (primary care physician) appointments at an FQHC (Federally Qualified Health Center) and intermittently attends AA (Alcoholics Anonymous) meetings. The palliative assessment was that the member needs structure and support. He does need regular PCP visits. Ideally, he should stop smoking and get permanent housing, but member not currently interested.

The palliative team arranged weekly visits at his car, at a senior center, or at other designated area. Phone call reminders were a key to providing structure and support. He was reminded of PCP appointments and to take his meds. His Friday "tuck in call" avoided weekend emergencies. The team continued discussion of housing and smoking and maintained phone contact.

No hospitalizations or ED visits occurred over 10 months. The patient is willing to talk to someone about permanent housing.

This case emphasizes the value of addressing social determinants of health through support and structure. Coming to the patient, gaining his trust, and being creative in providing support far outweighed the effect of the medical interventions.

## 12. Bad news conversations

Delivering bad news or discussing end of life issues is not always a pleasant event. The most common barriers to delivering bad news is:

- Fear of causing emotional harm to the patient
- Fear of taking away "hope"
- Focusing away from "cure" is perceived as failure
- No one taught us about this in medical or nursing school
- Bad news discussions take time
- The initial response may not be pleasant

Proceeding with planning cannot occur until you get through the emotions:

- It takes time, often more than one conversation
- There's lots of questions and explanations
- The medical plan needs to be coordinated with the medical team
- The support plan may require an extra layer of support from a multidisciplinary team
- Ongoing re-evaluations are frequent
- Knowledge helps overcome fear

Although no one likes to deliver bad news, it is an essential component of quality medical care and may be the most remembered event by the patient and family. You cannot proceed with planning unless your patient has been informed.

- You cannot make bad news good
- Bad news may be seen differently by the deliverer and the recipient … there is medical reality and there is patient expectation
- The initial reaction to bad news may not be pleasant e.g. anger, denial, depression, blame
- Addressing bad news is essential to doing realistic planning: medical as well as emotional, spiritual, and supportive.
- Ask how much detail the recipient would like
- Respect cultural preferences and social disparities
- Patients and families do have a right to meaningful informed consent

Show your concern:

- Right setting- private
- Right participants- decision makers
- No interruptions
- Eye level conversation

Basic techniques for the Bad News Conversation (Adapted from Baile, Buckman, Lenzi, et al., The Oncologist, 2000; 5: 302).

Validation- we respect your feelings.

> "Many other patients have had similar experiences"
> "I can understand how you felt that way"

"You were correct to feel that way"

Empathy- we care

"I'm sorry to have to tell you this"
"This is difficult for me"
"I can see how upsetting this is to you"

Probe further- we need to talk more

"Tell me more about it"
"Could you explain what you mean"
"Could you tell me what you are worried about"

Ask the patient to summarize what they heard.
Discuss next steps and follow up.

## 13. Helpful hints

Acceptance of palliative care has been a slow process. It can be time consuming and uncomfortable, despite its benefits. Some of the key factors in having a successful program include:

- Communication and coordination: Palliative care patients have all their usual health benefits plus the palliative team. They may also have a managed care health plan. All these entities must coordinate their efforts to care for this vulnerable population.

- Patient participation: Severe progressive disease is both a physical burden and an emotional burden. The patients' wishes must be respected, regardless of our own personal opinions. We want to listen to the patient and help them to express their preferences.

- Family consensus: Disagreements among family members can be another barrier to good decision making. Everyone should try to respect the patient's choices. The goal of the Advance Directive is to designate the agent who would have the final say if the patient cannot make his/her decision. Cultural factors should be respected.

- 24 phone access to palliative providers: Most palliative providers can take phone calls or do interventions after working hours. This facilitates interventions that can prevent hospitalizations or emergency room visits.

- Health plan contacts (as problem solvers, hands on, real time): The palliative team and the medical team may not be able to navigate the health plan system. The health plan needs to have live personnel to assist those teams on benefit related issues, identifying contracted providers, or issues requiring prior authorization.

- Compassion, Open Mind, Listen: Severe progressive disease and/or end of life are emotional times. We must always try to put ourselves in the shoes of our patients to give them the most effective and empathetic support that we can.
- Not always successful: Palliative interventions are not always successful. We can try to do our best, but outcomes can vary despite the best care.
- Community support: Patients may need support from community-based organizations. The palliative team can navigate patients to community resources, provided that those services exist and have been identified. We may successfully navigate the patient to what they need, but if that resource does not exist we have just "navigated them to nowhere."

## 14. The elevator speech

Trying to explain palliative care to someone within one to two minutes may not be easy, but here is an elevator speech. The two versions are similar, but one is written in prose, and one is in bullet point format. There are some variations between different palliative programs. The health plan may or may not provide a palliative care benefit. The program may or may not be offered at no cost. The health plan may or may not require prior authorization. The plan may or may not have its own palliative team to review referrals and serve as a liaison between the referring party, the palliative provider, and the patient. The referring party may have contact directly with the actual palliative provider. Not all palliative teams provide phone access or emergency service after hours.

Version 1: Palliative care is a service which may be provided by your insurance company usually at no cost to the member or doctor (check this since palliative care may or may not be a benefit). A team of physicians, nurses, social workers, and coordinators provide an extra layer of support to your members with severe progressive disease in need of symptom control, advance care planning, or psycho-social support. These are members who are frequently in the hospital or emergency room. The member retains all their normal health plan benefits which are coordinated between the doctors, the medical group, the health plan, and the palliative care provider. The palliative care providers usually have an after- hours call line (check this since some palliative care providers may not have an after- hours call line or provide services after-hours) and can provide services after hours. To make a referral, just complete the referral form, and fax or e-mail it to the health plan or palliative provider (the insurer may require prior authorization). For questions, just call the health plan palliative team (check that the plan does have its own palliative team). A contact list and referral form is attached. All referrals will be reviewed by health plan palliative medical directors. Palliative care is a program for the living… to provide the highest quality of life despite serious illness. Please remember that palliative care is not hospice. With palliative care the member may continue their disease focused treatment and there is no 6-month limitation. The palliative program has improved members' quality of life and reduced their usage of the hospital and emergency department to manage their illness. Our members and our doctors appreciate the extra layer of support that has been coordinated for them.

Version 2: Elevator speech in bullet point format.

- Our palliative care program is a home-based palliative care program (check if the program is either a clinic-based program or a telehealth program rather than home based.)
- Members are often scared off by the term "palliative care" because they confuse it with hospice
- Palliative care is NOT hospice: Palliative care is not just end of life, it does not have a 6- month limitation, the member retains all their health plan benefits, and members may continue with all their disease focused treatments while on their palliative care program
- Palliative care is for the living
- The member retains their PCP, their specialists, and their medical group.
- The health plan has a team of nurses who screen the referrals and assist in coordinating care (check that the health plan does have contacts who review referrals)
- Referrals can be made by sending a referral form to or calling the health plan
- The palliative care program (check this since palliative care may or may not be a benefit) is at no cost to the member or medical group or doctors
- Referrals must be approved by the health plan (check if this is a requirement)
- Criteria for referral include members with severe and progressive disease, in need of symptom control, advance care planning, or psycho-social support.

## 15. Final thoughts

"You can't control the wind, but you can adjust your sails." Yiddish Proverb

"Life is like riding a bicycle. To keep your balance, you must keep moving." Albert Einstein.

## Acknowledgements

The author wishes to acknowledge Dr. Tao Le for his input for this publication and his assistance as co-founder of the Health Net, Inc. Care Connections© palliative care program.

## Conflict of interest

The author declares no conflict of interest.

## Notes/thanks/other declarations

The author wishes to thank Carole Nathanson, R.N. and the Health Net palliative care nursing team for their dedication in developing the palliative care program. The author also wishes to thank LightBridge Hospice and Palliative Care, San Diego, California, USA for their collaboration in caring for the case study patients referenced in this publication.

## Author details

Marvin J. Gordon
Department of Medical Affairs, Health Net, Inc, Cypress, California, USA

*Address all correspondence to: marvingordonmd@cox.net

## References

[1] Online: Who.int. Available from: https://www.who.int/news-room/fact-sheets/detail/palliative-care)put

[2] Temel JS, Greer JA, Muzikansky A, et al. Early palliative care for patients with metastatic non–small-cell lung cancer. The New England Journal of Medicine. 2010;**363**:733-742

[3] California Department of Health Care Services, All-Plan Letter (CA DHCS APL 18-020 December 7, 2019)

[4] Gordon MJ, Le T, Lee EW, Gao E. Home palliative care savings. Journal of Palliative Medicine. 2022;**25**(4):591-595

[5] Cassel JB, Kerr KM, McClish DK, et al. Effect of a home-based palliative care program on healthcare use and costs. Journal of the American Geriatrics Society. 2016;**64**:2288-2295

**Chapter 7**

# Ethics in Palliative Care

*Delgersuren Gelegjamts, Khulan Gaalan and Batbagana Burenerdene*


## Abstract

The cases of ethical issues (new and unfamiliar daily circumstances) are increasing every day in palliative care services. The role of the codes of ethics is to help with these problems. The goal of end-of-life care for dying patients is to prevent or relieve suffering and respect the patient's wishes and values. The benefits of ethical decision-making are relief of pain, improving the patient's recovery, reducing the side effects of treatment, prevention of depression, and increasing quality of life. An essential component of the ethical decision-making processes may concern patients' family members and society. However, physicians, healthcare teams, and nurses are facing difficulties in ethical challenges in end-of-life care. It should also protect the patient's rights, dignity, beliefs, and religion. Healthcare professionals should understand the principles of ethics, ethical legal documents, advanced care planning, and ethical conflict to help patients make the best decision possible. The ethical principles guide healthcare professionals in the management of these situations and the problem they face in end of life care. In this chapter, we will cover the consideration regarding the ethical principles, ethical issues, ethical challenges, and dilemmas during the palliative care. The cases of ethical issues are increasing every day in the palliative care service.


**Keywords:** end-of-life care, ethics, advance directives, ethical dilemmas, decision-making

## 1. Introduction

Palliative care (PC) alleviates the distressing symptoms in a terminal stage of diseases, avoids harm of intention, and improves the quality of life (QOL). The goal of PC should be to let the patients maintain their dignity and hope while they are alive [1]. The PC team should be knowledgeable enough to provide appropriate care, respect patients, rights, and avoid conflicts [2]. It involves a multi-disciplinary team that provides medical care, pain management, and emotional and spiritual support to a person and family members [3]. The QOL of life of a cancer patient has a direct connection with the professional and nonprofessional caregiver's knowledge of supportive care and attitude toward end-of-life (EOL) care [4].

Many people at the EOL experience unnecessary difficulty and suffering [5]. Death is an inevitable part of life and death and should be peaceful, pain-free, and without any suffering [1]. Advanced medicine and modern technologies have both prolonged life expectancies and transformed the natural norms of death. Although, those new treatments and technologies do not cure chronic diseases. Medical interventions such as artificial nutrition and respiratory support can extend their life and provide secondary support [5].

The difficulties of ethical issues and moral solutions in palliative care services ethical principles recognized universally are autonomy, beneficence, non-maleficence, and justice [5]. A good understanding of medical ethics will contribute to the health professional's decision-making and the daily practice of medicine for EOL patients [2].

## 2. Palliative care and related ethics

### 2.1 Ethics of palliative care and hospices

Worldwide only about 14% of people who need PC currently receive it, and each year an estimated 56.8 million people, including 25.7 million in the last year of life, require palliative care [6]. The goal of the PC is to improve the QOL for both the patient and their family members. Many people have difficulties and suffering at the end of life EOL experience. EOL helps with anxiety and distressful emotions, such as fear of the future and being a burden to loved ones. They worry about pain management and the loss of control over the quality of their lives [7].

WHO: " PC is an improves the QOL of patient and family members facing the problems related with life-threatening illness, through the prevention and relief of suffering using of early identification and complete assessment and treatment of pain and other needs specially physical, psychosocial and spiritual" [8].

PC is a specialized medical care for people living with a serious illness [9]. Hospice and PC were established in the middle of the year 1900 and the founder who is Dame Cicely Saunders. She opened the first modern hospice (named St. Christopher Hospice-1965) and published a book about death (On Death and Dying-1969) [10].

PC improves the QOL of patients and their family members and most importantly is the reduction in symptoms of burden [11]. PC is explicitly recognized under the human right to health. It should be provided through person-centered and integrated health services that pay special attention to the specific needs and preferences of individuals [8]. Advancements in the development of medicine and technologies have both prolonged life expectancies and transformed the natural norms of death [5]. However, modern technologies and treatments do not cure chronic diseases, and medical intervention is providing secondary support such as artificial nutrition and respiratory support that can prolong lives [5, 12].

PC is specialized care provided to terminally ill patients by a multidisciplinary team. "Terminally ill" is defined as a patient who is affected by an incurable disease associated with a prognosis defined by an amount of months, days, or even hours of life. The multidisciplinary team is aimed to respect the dignity of human and improves their QOL, through pain control and relief of other symptoms.

PC is best for controlling the symptoms in these difficult situations [11] and focuses on the best quality of life for patients and family members [13]. Family members feel anger, blame, loss of hope, and weakness when they cannot relieve the suffering of their terminally ill loved one [14]. Terminally ill patients will have a hard time deciding because of sadness and stress [5]. The delivery of palliative services to patients and their loved ones should be managed in an ethical manner [6]. EOL is both a clinical and ethical challenge [15].

### 2.2 Ethics of healthcare team of palliative care

PC is provided by a specially trained team of doctors, nurses, and other specialists who work together with a patient's serious illness. PC is comprehensive, also interdisciplinary services [16], and total care concentrates primarily on the comfort and support of patients and families who has a serious illness like cancer, heart failure, advanced lung disease, and neurodegenerative disorders [17]. The team's palliative and supportive care is especially and serves them with holistic services including as emotional, spiritual, functional, and physical support. Healthcare professionals play crucial roles in the delivery of PC for cancer patients as they have to provide healthcare services with a positive attitude and also be prepared mentally [4].

Physicians and nurses face difficulties in their clinical practice of PC, and they need to understand ethical principles and standards well [2, 18] because health professionals need the right decision-making and the daily practice of medicine for terminally ill patients [19]. The PC experts and team members should carry out their responsibilities with honesty and dignity Palliative care, therefore, requires many different competencies, not only clinical but also relational, communicative, and ethical [20].

Essential skills needed for PC teams and clinicians who provide clinical care for EOL patients are education on medical ethics, understanding ethical principles, focusing on serious illness, learning about advanced care planning, ethics conflict, ethics committees, and specialist palliative care teams' goals [21].

Nursing as a profession was created by society to meet specific perceived health needs [13]. Their daily ethical challenges influence those factors as spiritual beliefs, religious practice, and cultural norms of the patient. The patient's culture like beliefs about disease treatment, and attitude affected their health and healing process [22].

The roles of the nurse are to work as a member of the interdisciplinary team so the patient/family can make fully informed decisions with full knowledge of the consequences of those options. In addition, PC nurses play a pivotal role in ethical issues.

Nurses are the most essential to the patients for ethical decision-making in PC because the nurses spend more time with patients and develop communication of intimacy and trust inherent in the nurse-patient relationship [14]. Andrew Jameton [23], a philosopher and author of nursing ethics, confidently states that "Nursing is the morally central health care profession". Ethical leadership in nursing requires fundamental nursing values such as respect for patients, harmless, and justice.

According to the international code of ethics for nurses by the International Council of Nurses (ICN) [24], nurses are responsible for promoting health, preventing illness, restoring health, and to alleviate suffering. Professional code of ethics states "consistent with existing professional codes of ethics, conflicts of interest, scopes of practice, and standard of care for all relevant disciplines [21], and both codes state that nurses should provide respectful and equitable care to all individuals, families, and communities needing nursing care regardless of age, color, creed, culture, disability or illness, gender, sexual orientation, nationality, politics, race, or social status [25]. The ethics of PC often conflicts with clinicians, nurses, other healthcare team members, patients, and family members about what constitutes care, particularly as death approaches [26]. Healthcare organizations can work toward developing and implementing guidelines & policies for EOL care decision-making, especially policies for withholding or withdrawing the treatment options so as to avoid ethical dilemmas.

### 2.3 Palliative care patients

PC is available to anyone regardless of age as long as they have been diagnosed with an illness that causes suffering or is untreatable such as cancer, multiple chronic conditions as long as the patient or family members need or who want to relieve their suffering. In any setting where patients receive EOL care such as a home, palliative units, hospice units, PC clinics, and nursing homes. A professional team provides clinical care. However, primary health services are possible with a family physician, internist, geriatrician, cardiologist, pulmonologist, intensivist, and nurses [3].

PC offers physical, emotional, social, and functional support to people who need end-of-life care. PC teams and especially nurses face death and take care of people who are affected by death regardless of the terminal illness and settings where they work [27]. However, most Asian patients like to spend their valuable time at home and with their family members. PC patients have to follow principles for decision-making in their own life.

1. Every adult has the right to decide for themselves. People are assumed to have the mental capacity to make decisions until it is proven otherwise.

2. People should be given every possible help before they are declared to not have the mental capacity. This includes different forms of communication such as blinking, movement, and making noises.

3. If someone makes a decision that seems unwise or strange, it does not mean they lack the mental capacity, and they have the right to make these decisions.

4. Any decision made on behalf of someone who lacks the mental capacity has to be made in their 'best interest".

5. People who lack mental capacity should not have their basic rights and freedom restricted, and any decision made on their behalf should not interfere with their rights or freedom.

## 3. Ethical issues and palliative care

Common ethics issues in PC include the goal of care, advanced directives issues, patient and family goal conflicts, physician and patient goal conflicts, transitioning focus of care, pain and symptom management, and PC and hospice treatment [3]. Most stressful ethical and patient care issues were protecting patients' rights, autonomy, and consent form to treatment, staffing patterns, and surrogate decision-making [28]. The staffing issues include physicians, nurses, teams, and volunteer [3]. The communication-related issues include the staff and patients/family members, physicians, patients, etc.

### 3.1 Ethics and moral attitudes palliative care profession

Moral philosophy is considered essential in moral issues, an important discussion about whether something is good or bad and right or wrong [14]. Ethics discipline is the study of the rational justification of moral principles and moral behavior [29].

Ethics is a process for making logical and consistent decisions based on social morality and philosophical reflection [14].

Both ethics issues and PC have always been a part of Medicine [11]. PC is a holistic approach, and ethical issues are an essential part of the principles of PC. The ethical principles and values in clinical practice refer to the importance of respecting all of a person's values, needs, and wishes in the context of health care, and that is the benefit to the person with an advanced chronic or terminal condition [30]. The morality of PC recognizes the moral principles; moral dimension, communication; and moral dilemmas as individual conflicts [31].

### 3.2 Ethical principles of palliative care

The principle was originally proposed by Beauchamp and Childress [32]. They included autonomy in the principles, beneficence, and justice. An ethical principle include: Autonomy (an individual has the freedom to make their personal choices), Beneficence (to do together, sharing knowledge and listening they thought), Non-maleficence (without harm to people), and Justice (to encourage honesty and equality in individual). These "four principles" are common in Eastern and Western cultures, but their application and weight may differ [5].

Autonomy is careful about a patient's right to independence. Everybody has the right to decide the differences of treatment they receive unless they are proven to be unable to. Patients' autonomy should be respected and is one of the fundamental principles of medical ethics [33].

The beneficence requires the patient's charge of choosing the needs and preferences of the patient's treatment options and care. These should be regularly reviewed; recognized and acted upon so the patient can live as comfortably as long as possible with their inalienable human dignity always respected [5].

Non-maleficence is an obligation not to inflict harm intentionally [21]. Non-maleficence is the most important principle out of the four guiding principles of ethical decision-making.

Justice requires that those who are ill and all other people involved in their care families, careers, and even the wider community are treated fairly and that limited resources are used responsibly and wisely. Additionally, dignity (the patients and the persons have to respect their dignity) and truthfulness and honesty (the concept of informed consent and truth-telling) [2].

## 4. Ethical challenge in palliative care

Schofield et al. [34] analyzed a systematic review of the ethical challenges in PC practices. The researchers identified the daily practice of the ethical challenge, and the ethical issues and problems related to ethical principles, delivery of clinical care, working with family members, navigating societal values and expectations, and philosophy of PC.

"Decision-making" for EOL care has earned paramount importance as it has capability to prolong the human life with the support of medical technologies or can let the natural death process continue by foregoing the treatment option [35].

Many of these dilemmas are associated with decisions made concerning continuing, limiting, or withdrawing life-sustaining treatments [36]. The ethical dilemmas surrounding the provision of patient care include clinical decision-making. Honest communication about the diagnosis and prognosis of a fatal illness, which fully respects patients' wishes and preferences, positively affects their QOL and improves symptom management [37].

### 4.1 Decision-making and ethical principles

Each principle relates to each of the other three principles; therefore, they should be ordered according to the criteria of priority for each case, with the ultimate aim of "the best interests of the patient". The patient who is in the PC unit should make decision about his/her treatment and services. The patient's ability of the person to choose and act for one's self free of controlling influences such as coercion from physician, nurse, consultant, family members, and pressure from religious groups. Ability to make decisions based upon our personal values and wishes [3]. Autonomy was highly respected in EOL care and decision-making Nurses communicated major concerns in considering patients' preferences, wishes, and promoting advance care planning [38]. Beneficence is acting in the best interest of the patients. That was the best-case scenario and worst-case scenario. In the best-case scenario, we help the patient understand what QOL is and respect their values. In the worst-case scenario, the nurse or person taking care of the patient treat the patient with paternalistic interactions and does not respect their beliefs and values [3]. Non-maleficence is an important requirement in morality and palliative care ethics (do not harm) [39] and make no knowing act or decision, or lack of information sharing which will cause direct harm to the patient [3].

Justice is considered an individual's decision of what is better for the better of the patients and society. These decisions impact more than our own personal sphere and are responsible for the health status of the community [3].

### 4.2 Communication and decision-making

Issues of communication involve disclosure, confidentiality, informed consent, and decisional capacity. The most common reasons are conflicts in values between physician and patient or patient and his family [1]. The decision-making process presented has important elements such as the patients have to understand relevant information about his/her problem, respecting their choices, personal and patient's benefit, and ability to reason and to deliberate about available choices [13]. A nurse is the key person in the decision-making process between physicians and patients or surrogates.

#### *4.2.1 Disclosure includes*

The patient's present medical condition, likely course of treatment or what might happen if no treatment, if provided potential treatments will that may help the patient in prolonging their life or saving them as well as their risks and reduce unwanted burden. A professional opinion is suggested to patients on alternative treatments and recommendations based on the professional best clinical judgment [40].

#### *4.2.2 Confidentiality*

Sensitive personal information disclosed by a patient to their nurses is legally guarded by confidentiality, and should not be divulged and the necessary steps to ensure it should be taken [40]. The confidential information should be applied to non-autonomous and deceased patients as well. The only exception to this is if it is used to avoid harm in any way possible to either the patient or a third party [41].

#### *4.2.3 Informed consent*

When a patient goes to the health profession for a medical problem, the health profession is expected to make a diagnosis, inform them of all possible treatments and recommend one of them explaining the reason its pros and cons so they can make the most informed choice and express a preference for one of the suggested options given. The patient must understand the information, consider the treatment choices, and expresses a preference for one of the options planned by the physicians. This denotes the practical use of respect for the patient's autonomy [40].

#### *4.2.4 Decisional capacity*

The patient can make their own decision unless proven that they cannot. The patient should be able to understand relevant information, the medical situation; possible risks communicate a choice even if it is as small as a nod or the shake of a head as well as engage in relation deliberation with their values in the recommended treatment [40]. The patients have a right to refuse to make a decision and refer the decision-making process to another person.

## 5. Ethics dilemmas in palliative care patients

### 5.1 Dilemmas of ethics

Ethical dilemmas on macro- and micro-levels emerge daily as the debate continues on extending life versus postponing death [20]. Changes in social/family systems have added to the complexity of EOL and PC [15]. Ethical dilemmas surface as those comparisons draw attention to the insufficiencies of practice. For an ethics standard to be meaningful, it must reflect a comprehensive approach that simultaneously allows for each individual's particular needs. The extraordinary spectrum of requisites, from the most basic of physical care concerns to the broad issues of existential distress, reflects the daunting ethical responsibilities which are integral to PC. Ferrell's QOL model, which identifies the essential components of physical, psychological, social, and spiritual well-being, is comprehensively reflected in the Five Principles of PC. These principles can serve as a "checklist" for any healthcare professional caring for persons at the EOL.

Ethical dilemmas emerge across the spectrum of care as nurses endeavor to provide the best possible physical and psychological care, communicate appropriately and honestly with the patient and families in making decisions to withhold or withdraw treatment, and respond to requests for interventions that may conflict with their value systems [42]. Medical professional obligations are confidentiality, advance directives, DNAR, euthanasia and PAS, research, patient competence, "right to die," and power of attorney [41].

### 5.2 Advanced care planning

Advanced care planning (ACP) is a process that helps patients in any stage of health in understanding and share their values, life goals [43], and preferences and wishes regarding future treatments [44]. Substituted judgment refers to a guide for decision-making when a patient has difficulty decision-making and doctors, nurses, and family members try to make the decision that the patient would have made if his/her were able to make decisions [42]. ACP involves identifying a surrogate decision-maker to action if the patient is no longer able to make decisions about their care [45]. Surrogate decision-makers try to understand the patient's beliefs and values on the patient's behalf [21].

ACP is dependent on the patients' health whether they have a mild, or moderate chronic illness or advanced life-threatening [29]. ACP should be integrated into routine care and should be discussed frequently and every time the patient's condition changes [45].

The principle of the advanced care planning approach is commonly used for patients who are close to death to discuss with them about their future care and how they wish to be treated. However, these processes are not always been done, especially if; the patient is urgently admitted to the hospital or disagreement among family members about what is appropriate treatment [46].

Honoring Choices North Dakota (HCND) is defined as "Advance Directives are legal documents that allow patients to put their healthcare wishes in writing or to appoint someone they trust to make decisions for them if they become incapacitated" [21]. Types of advance directive names have Living will, personal directive, medical directive, advance decision, and mental health advance directive types of health care agent names are medical power of attorney (POA), health care power attorney, health care representative, health care surrogate, surrogate decision maker, and guardian and conservator [21].

### 5.3 Euthanasia and physician-assisted dying

Euthanasia on the conflicting can be both passive and active. Passive euthanasia mentions to hastening the death of an individual by taking away a form of support and agreeing for the patient to die naturally without support; active euthanasia is affecting the death of someone through direct action at an individual's request. Proponents claim that the suffering, anguish, and pain of the patient and family could be more. Finally, the public, individuals, families, and healthcare providers need to openly and honestly discuss all aspects of this approach to disease management at the end of life [7]. As of 2022, euthanasia is legal in Belgium, Canada, Colombia, Luxembourg, the Netherlands, New Zealand, Spain, and several states of Australia (New South Wales, Queensland, South Australia, Tasmania, Victoria, and Western Australia) and seven states in the US (Wikipedia, 2022). PAD is an ethical argument regarding voluntary euthanasia and it is from a utilitarian perspective [47].

### 5.4 Death

Professor Alexander Fitzthum [48] recorded that death is classified into five groups, natural, accidental, suicidal, homicide, and unknown death. Natural death is an internal factor that causes the body to shut down (chronic diseases such as cancer, heart diseases, diabetics.) and an external factor such as traumatic injuries.

Many physicians, particularly those in the fields of oncology and PC, will be faced with a request for such assistance sometime in their professional lifetimes. In recent years, much of the developed world has seen the emergence of EOL debates and increasing pressures for the legalization of physician-assisted dying (PAD). It is challenging because of the inherent uncertainty of making predictions and because dying is not an easy topic to discuss [49].

Physician-assisted dying in utilitarian theory is considered ethically right as its decision is in the interest of the patient. Their family's interest should not be included and they should only be allowed to give their opinion on the patient's choice [9].

From the perspectives of patients, there is considerable debate regarding the ethical implications of physician-assisted dying; the patient's self-determination rights, competence, beliefs, and values form the basis for these decisions [9]. The physician-assisted death is a more respectful and dignified way for terminally ill patients to die. Most people including physicians agree with physician-assisted death; however, there is a need for training, support, and implementation of physician-assisted death. Ethics committees may help fill this gap and provide resources and mediation of value conflicts [9].

## 6. Conclusion

The conclusion of this chapter is palliative care is to prevent or relieve suffering available while respecting end-of-life patients. Ethical issues in palliative care increasing day-to-day in clinical care due to modern therapy and technology, and it is making life expectancies to increase. Healthcare professionals face difficult ethical challenges in daily work. The most important part of professional ethic appears to be communication, decision-making process, consent form, and ethical conflicts. Healthcare professionals should understand ethical principles, bioethical codes, legal documents, and end-of-life care. These can be prevented from ethical conflicts and ethical problems.

## Author details

Delgersuren Gelegjamts[1,2]*, Khulan Gaalan[3] and Batbagana Burenerdene[4]

1 Chosun University, South Korea

2 Mongolian National University, Mongolia

3 Mongolian National University of Medical Sciences, Mongolia

4 Seojeong College, Yanju, South Korea

*Address all correspondence to: degijulie@gmail.com

## References

[1] Rastogi P. Ethics in palliative care. In: Cascella M, editor. Highlights on Several Underestimated Topics in Palliative Care. London: IntechOpen; 2017. DOI: 10.5772/intechopen.70508

[2] Mohanti BK. Ethics in palliative care. Indian Journal of Palliative Care. 2009;**15**(2):89-92. DOI: 10.4103/0973-1075.58450

[3] Barb Supanich. Ethical issues in palliative care nursing. PowerPoint PPT Presentation. 2008

[4] Gelegjamts D, Burenerdene B. Supportive and palliative care attitude for cancer patients. Supportive and Palliative Care and Quality of Life in Oncology. 2023. DOI: 10.5772/intechopen.104757

[5] Akdeniz M et al. Ethical considerations at the end-of-life care. SAGE Open Medicine. 2021;**9**:12. DOI: 10.1177/20503121211000918

[6] Word Health Organization. 2022. Available from: https://www.who.int/

[7] McKinnon B, Orellana-Barrios M. Ethics in physician-assisted dying and euthanasia. The Chronicles. 2019;**7**(30):36-42. Available from: https://pulmonarychronicles.com/index.php/pulmonarychronicles/article/view/561

[8] Word Health Organization. 2020. Available from: https://www.who.int/

[9] Available from: https://www.capc.org/about/palliative-care/

[10] Macauley RC. Ethics in Palliative Care: A Complete Guide. Oxford University Press; 2018

[11] Steigleder T, Kollmar R, Ostgathe C. Palliative care for stroke patients and their families: barriers for implementation. Frontiers in Neurology. 2019;**10**:164

[12] Karnik S, Kanekar A. Ethical issues surrounding end-of-life care: A narrative review. Healthcare. 2016;**4**(2):24

[13] Burkhardt MA, Nathaniel A. Ethics and Issues in Contemporary Nursing. Cengage Learning; 2013

[14] Crane MK, Wittink M, Doukas DJ. Respecting end-of-life treatment preferences. American Family Physician. 2005;**72**(7):1263-1268

[15] Myers J, Shetty N. Going beyond efficacy: Strategies for cancer pain management. Current Oncology. 2008;**15**:8-9

[16] Hui D, Kim SH, Kwon JH, Tanco KC, Zhang T, Kang JH, et al. Access to palliative care among patients treated at a comprehensive cancer center. The Oncologist. 2012;**17**(12):1574-1580

[17] ANA. Available from: http://www.nursingworld.org

[18] Beauchamp TL, Childress JF. Principles of Biomedical Ethics. Edicoes Loyola; 1994

[19] Fins J. A Palliative Ethic of Care: Clinical Wisdom at life's End. Jones & Bartlett Learning; 2006

[20] Sepúlveda C, Marlin A, Yoshida T, et al. Palliative care: The World Health Organization's global perspective. Journal of Pain and Symptom Management. 2002;**24**(2):91-96. DOI: 10.1016/S0885-3924(02)00440-2

[21] Nancy Joyner. Legal and ethical Aspects of Palliative care: Addressing

Consent and Decision-Making challenge. 2022. Available from: https://ruralhealth.und.edu/.../palliative-care-ethics.pdf

[22] Vaughn LM, Jacquez F, Bakar RC. Cultural health attributions, beliefs, and practices: Effects on healthcare and medical education. The Open Medical Education Journal. 2009;**2**(1)

[23] Review: [Untitled]." Business & Professional Ethics Journal 4, no. 1. 1985. DOI: 10.2307/27799853 [Accessed March 17, 2023]

[24] Stievano A, Tschudin V. The ICN code of ethics for nurses: A time for revision. International Nursing Review. 2019;**66**(2):154-156

[25] Okada H. Japanese. Journal of the International Phonetic Association. 1991;**21**(2):94-96

[26] Eric K Fromme, Robert M Arnold, Jane Givens. Ethical issues in Palliative care. 2022. www.uptodate.com

[27] Izumi S, Nagae H, Sakurai C, Imamura E. Defining end-of-life care from perspectives of nursing ethics. Nursing Ethics. 2012;**19**(5):608-618. DOI: 10.1177/0969733011436205

[28] Ulrich CM, Taylor C, Soeken K, O'Donnell P, Farrar A, Danis M, et al. Everyday ethics: ethical issues and stress in nursing practice. Journal of Advanced Nursing. 2010;**66**(11):2510-2519. DOI: 10.1111/j.1365-2648.2010.05425

[29] Cambridge dictionary

[30] Barrocas A, Geppert C, Durfee SM, Maillet JO, Monturo C, Mueller C, et al. ASPEN ethics position paper. Nutrition in Clinical Practice. 2010;**25**(6):672

[31] De Panfilis L, Di Leo S, Peruselli C, Ghirotto L, Tanzi S. "I go into crisis when ...": Ethics of care and moral dilemmas in palliative care. BMC Palliative Care. 2019;**18**(1):70. DOI: 10.1186/s12904-019-0453-2

[32] Beachaump T, Childress J. Principles of Biomedical Ethics. Seventh ed. Oxford: Oxford University Press; 2012

[33] Andorno R. The right not to know: An autonomy-based approach. Journal of Medical Ethics. 2004;**30**(5):435-439

[34] Schofield G, Dittborn M, Huxtable R, Brangan E, Selman LE. Real-world ethics in palliative care: A systematic review of the ethical challenges reported by specialist palliative care practitioners in their clinical practice. Palliative Medicine. 2021;**35**(2):315-334. DOI: 10.1177/0269216320974277

[35] Meisel A. From birth to death and bench to clinic: The Hastings center bioethics briefing book for journalists, policymakers, and campaigns. In: Crowley M, editor. End-of-Life Care. Garrison the Hastings Center: Garrison, NY, USA; 2008. pp. 51-54

[36] Wiegand DL, MacMillan J, dos Santos MR, Bousso RS. Palliative and end-of-life ethical dilemmas in the intensive care unit. AACN Advanced Critical Care. 2015;**26**(2):142-150

[37] Back AL, Anderson WG, Bunch L, et al. Communication about cancer near the end of life. Cancer. 2008;**113**(7 Suppl):1897-1910. DOI: 10.1002/cncr.23653

[38] Hernández-Marrero P, Fradique E, Pereira SM. Palliative care nursing involvement in end-of-life decision-making: Qualitative secondary analysis. Nursing Ethics. 2019;**26**(6):1680-1695. DOI: 10.1177/0969733018774610

[39] Al-Bar MA, Chamsi-Pasha H. Contemporary Bioethics: Islamic Perspective. Cham (CH): Springer; 2015

[40] Jonsen A, Siegler M, Winslade W. Clinical Ethics. New York, NY: Mc Graw-Hill; 2002

[41] Randall F, Downie RS. 'Confidentiality', Palliative Care Ethics: A Companion for All Specialties, 2nd edn (Oxford, 1999; online edn, Oxford Academic, 17 Nov. 2011), [Accessed 21 Mar. 2023]

[42] Betty R. Ferrell and Nessa Coyle Palliative Nursing Book. 2nd ed. 2006

[43] Beauchamp TL. Philosophical Ethics. 3th ed. Boston: McGraw-Hill; 2001

[44] Derek D. Guidelines and Suggestions for those Starting a Hospice/Palliative Care Service. 3th ed. Houston: IAHPC Press; 2021

[45] Torke AM, Alexander GC, Lantos J. Substituted judgment: the limitations of autonomy in surrogate decision making. Journal of General International Medicine. 2008;**23**(9):1514-1517. DOI: 10.1007/s11606-008-0688-8

[46] Sudore RL, Lum HD, You JJ, et al. Defining advance care planning for adults: A consensus definition from a multidisciplinary Delphi panel. Journal of Pain and Symptom Management. 2017;**53**:821

[47] Singer P. Voluntary euthanasia: A utilitarian perspective. Bioethics. 2003;**17**(5-6):526-541

[48] Alexander F. Death is usually considered "natural" if it wasn't caused by an external factor. 22 Feb 2022. Available from: https://health.osu.edu/authors/alexander-fitzthum-md

[49] Steinhauser KE, Tulsky JA. Defining a 'good' death. In: Cherny N, Fallon M, Kaasa S, Portenoy RK, editors. Oxford Textbook of Palliative Medicine. edn ed. Currow DC: Oxford University Press; 2015

Chapter 8

# Advances in Burn Care in Hong Kong: Reflecting on a Decade of Expert Experiences from Local Practice with an International Perspective

*Tze-Wing Wong, Ka-Huen Yip, Yuk-Chiu Yip and Wai-King Tsui*

## Abstract

The nursing implications of burn injuries extend beyond the immediate health concerns over the loss of skin integrity, the presence of scarring, and the psychological impacts on patients due to disfigurement. Non-fatal burns may lead to long-term disabilities, hence advanced nursing care may be required to prevent such outcomes. In Hong Kong, advances have been made to ensure that sophisticated nursing services and care are in place for affected patients. This chapter discusses how burn injuries are managed at different levels within a publicly funded acute care framework, explains how professional competencies regarding burn care are developed among burn care nurses, delineates the roles of medical technology in supporting wound assessment, explains the application of novel dressing materials for various burn wound conditions, and outlines how the establishment of nurse-led clinics can promote the continuity of care for patients with burn injuries. Written with an international perspective with the authors' practice experiences in Hong Kong (China), this chapter provides evidence-based reference for registered nurses in general, specialty nurses, nurse practitioners, and nurse consultants worldwide.

**Keywords:** burn care, burn care team, burn care nurses, nurse-led clinic, medical technology in burn care

## 1. Introduction

Burn injuries are life-threatening and cause significant functional and cosmetic morbidity [1, 2]. Managing patients with burn injuries remains challenging, particularly in severe cases [3].

The most common are scald burn injuries that occur in home settings [4]. Toddlers and children are accidentally scalded by hot fluids due to the carelessness of parents and caregivers [5]. Furthermore, most burns in older adults occur at home since they stay alone, are more prone to medical comorbidities, and are at high risk for burn and scald injury [6–9]. Nevertheless, over the past decade, significant advances in training and development, burn wound assessment, burn wound closure technologies, and continuity of follow-up have been made [10–12].

## 2. How burn injuries are managed at different levels within a publicly funded acute care framework

In Hong Kong, under the governance of the Hospital Authority in the acute burn care framework, patients with burn injuries are managed in hospitals with recognized standards and trained specialty healthcare professionals [13–15]. This organizational structure provides a more coordinated care by centralizing patients with severe burn injuries, thereby facilitating the delivery of quality medical and nursing services and early transfer to a burn unit/facility. There remains no universal naming criteria as to what qualifies burn treatment premises to be "burn unit" or "burn facility"; hence, in this chapter, we follow the existing terms of the current treatment premises determined by the Hospital Authority, which is the central governance body of all publicly funded hospitals in Hong Kong. In Hong Kong, some burn units are a major acute hospital among a cluster of regional hospitals caring for patients with major burn injuries, while burn facilities care for patients with moderate sized of burn injuries. According to the severity degree of burn injuries, burn surgeons in accident and emergency unit transfer patients to burn unit or burn facility following consultation when burn injuries meet the referral criteria (**Figure 1**) [15, 16].

Healthcare professionals including burn surgeons, nurses, physiotherapists, and occupational therapists deliver rehabilitation interventions such as medical treatment, therapy, or care for patients with minor burns categorized as Level 1. These patients are stabilized in general surgical or orthopedic units in different hospitals with designated facilities and healthcare professionals with the support of the

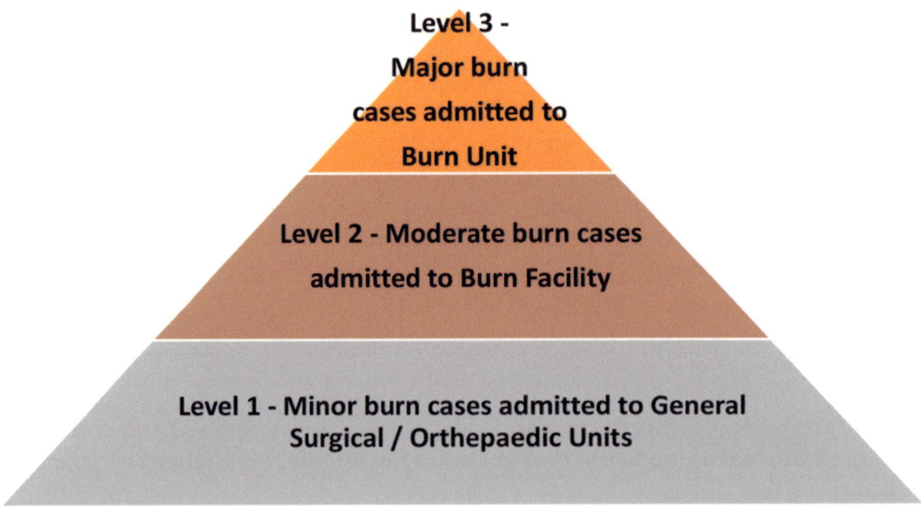


**Figure 1.**
*Networking of burn Service in Hong Kong.*

| |
|---|
| • Burns greater than 5% of total body surface area |
| • Burns that involve and threaten functional or cosmetic impairment of the face, hands, feet, genitalia, perineum, and major joints |
| • Full-thickness burns |
| • Electrical burns |
| • Chemical burns |
| • Circumferential burns of the limbs and chest |
| • Burns at the age-specific considerations (such as children and those age > 60 years old) |
| • Burns in patients with pre-existing medical conditions, which could complicate management, prolong recovery, or affect mortality |
| • Inhalation injury without skin involvement is excluded |

**Table 1.**
*Burn facility referral criteria at level 2.*

multidisciplinary team. In Hong Kong, senior burn surgeons act as the directors of the receiving burn units/facilities and coordinate the transfer management for all exposures of vulnerable populations to further risks in burns injuries. At the accident and emergency unit, patients with burn injuries are stabilized prior to transfer to the burn/facility to optimize the quality of care and treatment. Moderate-sized or complex burn injuries categorized as Level 2 are managed in a burn facility (**Table 1**) [17–19]. In Hong Kong, there are 3 burn facilities that care for patients namely Queen Elizabeth, Kwong Wah, and Tuen Mun Hospitals.

Patients with extensive and complicated burn injuries are categorized as Level 3 (**Table 2**) and managed or transferred to the burn unit [13, 17–19]. There are 2 burn units considered as the major acute hospital among a cluster of regional hospitals caring for patients with major burn injuries in Hong Kong. However, immediate resuscitation and intensive care support are mandatory. Therefore, optimal treatment of patients with extensive burn injuries requires advanced healthcare resources, implementation of multidisciplinary acute care collaboration, and planning for long-term rehabilitation.

### 2.1 Enhancing professional competencies regarding burn care are developed among burn care nurses

James et al. have previously reported a total of 8,991,468 patients with burn injuries in 195 countries and territories from 1990 to 2017 [20]. Previous studies have also reported that an estimated 180,000 deaths annually are attributed to burn injuries combined with electrical injuries, structural collapse, fire escape, airplane

| |
|---|
| • Burns greater than 20% and 10% of total body surface area for adult patients and children ≦12 years old, respectively |
| • Burns with major functional and/or cosmetic implications |
| • Burns in patients with significant pre-existing medical conditions that could complicate management, prolong recovery, or affect mortality |
| • Inhalation injury without skin damaged is excluded |

**Table 2.**
*Burn unit referral criteria at level 3.*

crashes, scald burns during assaults, and explosions with airborne flames [21–26]. At the global level, the age-standardized mortality due to burn injuries has significantly decreased from 1990 to 2017; only 3 out of 21 regions reported a significant increase in the incidence rates of burn injuries, and delineated rising rates by more than 30% of age-standardized incidence rates especially in China [20]. The reported indicated that most middle- and high-income regions have invested in resources and safety measures and established access to care to reduce/combat incidence of burn injuries.

A comprehensive burn team approach is important when providing burn care to patients with burn injury by burn care nurses with multidisciplinary care; a burn team consists of burn surgeons, nurses, physiotherapists, occupational therapists, dietitians, and psychologists [10, 27]. Burn care nurses play a crucial role in caring for patients with extensive burns [28] and disaster management, mainly in handling patients with burn injuries [29]. Competency-driven, high-quality, and evidence-based education training programs related to burn injuries are essential when preparing nurses for the full continuum of burn care management [30–32]. The number of burn nursing education and training programs has gradually expanded over the past 20 years [33]. Therefore, most existing training programs in Hong Kong focus on burns injuries management comprise preparedness, response, and recovery phases. Furthermore, most nurse training programs related to burns injuries, especially those targeting registered nurses, have adopted different teaching approaches (online and face-to-face) to ensure flexibility in time, location, and cost effectiveness [34, 35].

In the United States, different burn centers incorporate competencies within the educational nursing curriculums of training programs with examination aligned with the American Burn Association burn nurse competencies (BNC) [36]. Training programs establish interactive, evidenced-based, comprehensive, preceptor workshop, online learning, and skill practice module consistent with BNC domains. Domains of BNC consist of wound management, and other relevant supports (psychosocial, nutritional, discharge planning, and aftercare) [36].

Meanwhile, in the United Kingdom, registered nurses must complete specific burn courses and be competent in burn care by the end of their second year in burn centers and units [37, 38]. According to the framework of burn care for a burn-injured patient, training programs align with the National Burn Care Standards, and nurses require to attend an accredited course in the emergency management for severe burn [37, 38]. Moreover, lead nurses for the Burn Care Services must complete a specific burn care course to demonstrate competences and require attending burn specific training programs annually [38].

In Hong Kong, registered nurses with three-year experience are considered burn care nurses in different public hospitals and must complete an emergency management of severe burns course [13, 15]. Continuing professional education is vital for the future role of burn care nurses. However, to advance their practice, the *"Post-Registration Certificate Course in Advanced Surgical Nursing"* and *"Post-Registration Certificate Course in Burn and Plastic Surgical Nursing (PRCC in Burn & Plastic)"* are training programs recommend for burn care nurses to increase their competence in burn care nursing and facilitate the development of burn teams in a burn unit to meet the complexity of managing different levels of burn injuries by in-service training in Hong Kong [15].

*"Post-Registration Certificate Course in Advanced Surgical Nursing"* is an annual training program consisting of different surgical nursing specialties components (breast, urological, stoma and wound, hepatobiliary and pancreatic, head and neck and plastic, and burn and plastic care) with theoretical and practical components.

According to the burn patient population, conduction of *PRCC in Burn and Plastic* is affected by the demand of clinical services (e.g., held in 1997, 2016, and 2019). This program is an 8-month structured training program with examination. The core content of this program emphasizes the theoretical (210 lecture hours) and practical (6 weeks practical attachment) components to enhance the knowledge of burn care nurses in delivering burns nursing interventions [39]. Currently, becoming an experienced burn care nurse requires being a nursing burn team leader that helps to facilitate patients with burn injuries to the optimal level of physical and psychological health and social function [40]. The effect of stimulation training on the development of burn care nurses can positively affect the perceptions of nurses managing patients with burns injuries [32, 41]. The advancement of burn education through simulation training tools aimed at the emerging role of simulation for training to promote knowledge and significantly advance the delivery of burn education. It is crucial for competence enhancement of burn care nurses, such as providing experience with rare and critical incidents, problem-solving skills, decision-making, and team dynamics [13, 42–44]. Debriefing sessions during the simulation training program are critical for nursing education since they provide the opportunity for self-recall and insight into improving learning outcomes (critical analysis and personal growth) following simulation training workshops. This program can enhance the clinical skills critical in assisting new burn care nurses in their transition to practice.

Given the increased occurrence of disasters, including burns injuries, enhancing the readiness of burn care nurses caring for the physical and psychological health of patients is urgently needed [35].

To sustain the standard and competence of clinical practice, *"Advanced Nursing Standards and Specialty Nursing Practice Guidelines"* related to burn and plastic surgical nursing have been adopted in public hospitals and are regularly developed for burn care nurses to enhance their comprehensive knowledge and skills, as well as the guidelines in the whole spectrum of burns injuries management in Hong Kong [15]. All standards and guidelines for advanced nursing practices are designed to support evidence-based practices to ensure the quality and appropriate pathway for nursing professionals to meet the burn injuries challenges [32].

Caring for patients with burn injuries certainly requires teamwork both within and outside the hospital. However, nursing colleges developed a platform between burn care nurses and other health professionals useful for sharing the knowledge and experience of caring for this unique group of patients (such as introduction and elementary understanding of basic burn knowledge and wound dressing technique), thereby reinforcing the roles and functioning of burn care nurses. In Hong Kong, such a network exists; the Hong Kong College of Surgical Nursing (HKCSN) facilitates networking among local surgical professionals and is a good support source. Serving as a platform for healthcare professionals to share experiences in burns nursing, the HKCSN invites both local and international experts to deliver lectures and run courses and seminars for its members [45].

Burn care nurses frequently attend different faculty/organizational development conferences, both local and international, e.g., Burn and Plastic Forums organized by local burn unit and burn facilities and International Burn Conferences and Annual Scientific Meetings organized overseas [13, 15, 46]. These conferences help burn care nurses caring for patients with burn injuries to learn new strategies and information regarding the global insight of nursing education and practices on burn management. In addition, conferences have been held on the ability of nursing professionals to transfer new knowledge into their nursing practices for patients with burn injuries in clinical settings. Knowledge transfer may benefit from a better understanding of professional development related to burn care in clinical settings [47], which includes best practices in non-boundary burn and plastic specialty, advanced technology in burn care, and wound dressing techniques that can be integrated into local practice.

## 2.2 Roles of medical technology in supporting wound assessment

Patients with burn injuries benefit from early wound closure with local treatment consisting of cleansing, debridement, and routine burn wound dressing changes to minimize or control infection and improve wound healing [48, 49]. However, at the early stages of injury, it may be difficult to accurately define the depth of burn wounds. In Hong Kong, burn care nurses use laser Doppler imaging (LDI) (**Figure 2**) with non-invasive and non-contact devices for more accurate assessments that deliver a two-dimensional image of the burn area as an early objective determination of wound depth (depth analysis of the dermal circulation).

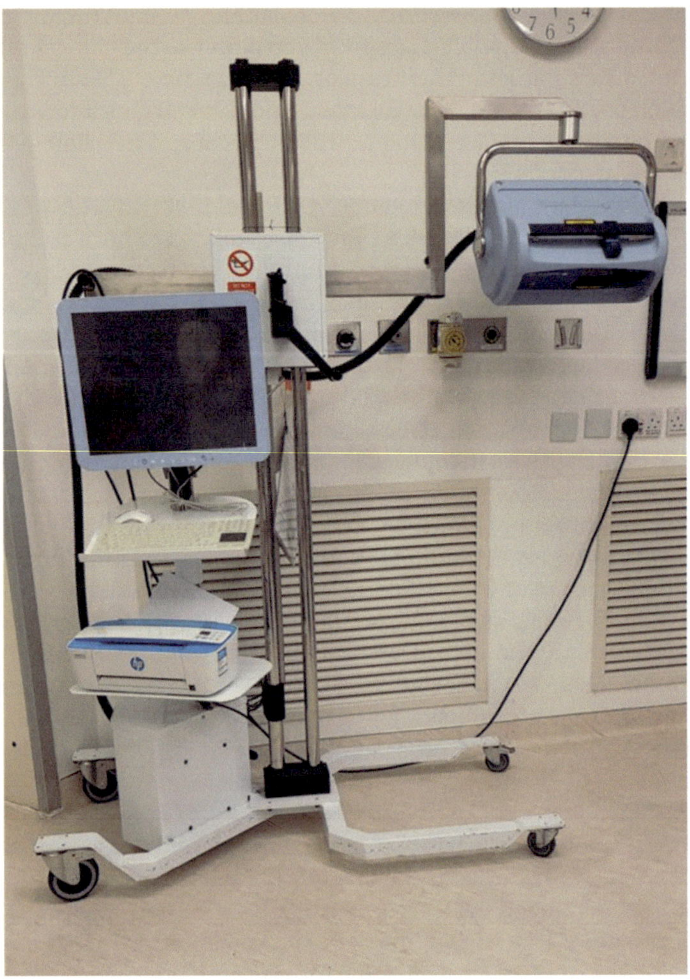

**Figure 2.**
*Laser Doppler imaging device.*

This technique also helps to predict the healing outcome of burn wounds before providing initial burn patient management [50–53], while the wound depth assessment is commonly determined and diagnosed by experienced burn surgeons using this imaging technique. This diagnostic intervention can be performed on patients with burns; hence wounds can be assessed early, between 48 hours to 5 days post-burn for diagnostic and therapeutic management [49, 52, 54].

There is a mandatory requirement to complete the LDI training qualification, which provides assessment knowledge and application skill essential for nursing clinicians in using this technique for therapeutic decisions for patients with burn injuries [51, 52, 54]. The completion requirement in operating LDI includes scanning technique, interpretation of results, awareness of safety practice, and elimination of confounding factors, including the presence of infection or tattoos [53–56]. However, the low power of the LDI laser light can penetrate the burn wound and detect circulating blood cells in capillaries, arterioles, and venules [49, 52, 55]. Moreover, LDI can identify a color-coded blood flow map showing microcirculatory blood perfusion in patients with burn injuries. LDI can differentiate superficial dermal burns, mid to deep dermal burns, and full-thickness burn wounds [51]. The utilization of LDI provides an early accurate assessment, thereby facilitating early burn treatment strategies, which can reduce costs, patient morbidity, length of hospitalization, and unnecessary surgery for patients with burns [55].

### 2.3 Application of novel dressing materials for various burn wound conditions

Burn care nurses perform routine burn wound dressing changes for patients with burn injuries, and their healing outcomes have been previously reviewed [48, 50, 57]. Burns can be classified by the depth of injury into either superficial, superficial dermal, deep dermal, full-thickness, and deeper injury [58–60]. According to the depth of the burn, various specialized management and treatment modalities are available and focus on specific anatomic sites; different therapeutic wound dressing materials are applied for the recovery of the underlying physiological processes in tissue repair such as antimicrobial agents, including gauze, non-adherent films, and antimicrobial agents [39, 61, 62]. The selection and application of dressing materials and topical agents are based on the nature of and benefits to the burn wound, a specific wound quality or presence of contamination or infection, and patient allergy.

Superficial burn wounds comprise superficial dermal and partial-thickness wounds that are pinkish in color, with blister formation, epidermis slough off, and excruciating pain [63]. Wound care promotes wound epithelialization and prevents infection. Furthermore, biological dressings, including porcine skin and amniotic membrane, are applied to relieve wound pain and enhance epithelialization [62, 63].

Deep burn wounds consist of deep partial thickness, full thickness, and deeper injury, and require burn wound excision and graft coverage. Mid- and deep-dermal burn wounds are mottled pinkish or whitish, have a dull sensation, and are sloughy [63]. The aims of wound care for deep burn wounds are minimizing necrotic tissue and preventing wound infection. First, wound irrigating disinfectant (e.g., Granudacyn® irrigation solution) is used to cleanse and moisturize the wound; it contains hypochlorous acid, a reliable cleansing solution [64] and can prevent the proliferation of Gram-positive and -negative bacteria. Subsequently, nurses should thoroughly cleanse and debride sloughy and necrotic tissue on a burn wound. A single-use sterile cloth, "UCS® debridement cloth", is pre-moistened and used for wound cleansing and debridement of the surrounding wound areas. Furthermore, enzymatic debridement agents (e.g., Iruxol® mono ointment dressing) are used to remove slough and promote burn wound healing and achieving a significant therapeutic effect [13].

Moreover, full-thickness burn wounds require eschar debridement and/or excision and original autologous meshed skin grafting for charred and leathery wound [63]. The use of skin grafts on full-thickness burn wounds results in no or minimum hypertrophic scar formation [65]. Simultaneously, burn care nurses require additional knowledge and skills to care for patients with burn injuries and guide the appropriate care of both the recipient (burn area with skin graft) and donor sites (donation skin site) [66].

### 2.4 Advancement of wound management for preventing hypertrophic scarring

Biodegradable temporizing matrix (BTM) is used for full or deep burn wounds [67–69] to cover excised deep burn wounds for at least 3 weeks, aiming at temporary wound closure and supporting the reconstruction of the dermis. BTM intergradation into the wound bed through cellular infiltration is time consuming. New blood vessels grow and become full of fibroblasts production; therefore, when the neodermis becomes vascularized, a thin skin graft can be applied to a deep burn wound [67, 70].

Dermal regeneration templates (e.g., Nevelia®) used for full or deep burn wounds or reconstructive surgery are made for collagen layering, which promotes dermal regeneration [71, 72]. First, it is used to cover an excised burn wound or excised scarring for approximately 3 weeks [73] and consists of a matrix of bovine collagen, which facilitates integration into the wound tissue [74]. Next, a split-thickness skin graft is required to cover burn wounds, provides better functional and esthetic outcomes, and reduces hypertrophic scar formation [65, 75].

### 2.5 Nurse-led burn clinics promote continuity of care for patients with burn injuries

Hong Kong has only one nurse-led burn clinic in public hospital, which plays a crucial role for patients with burn injuries by function-limiting sequelae such as contractures, scarring, thermoregulatory anomalies, amputation, and nurse-led burn clinic by promoting the continuity of care, quality of life, and psychosocial well-being during their rehabilitation and return home within the long-term recovery period, and by decreasing the length of hospitalization [39]. The aims of nurse-led burn clinics include: independent burn care nurses with delegated authority to make decisions regarding patients with burn injuries; delivering full support while maintaining continuity of care after discharge; implementation of multidisciplinary acute care collaboration and planning for long term rehabilitation and burn wound management; evaluating the patient's response to both physical and psychological treatments and counseling; referring the patient to the appropriate resources for support; assessing and evaluating the patient's ability to perform activities of daily living and self-care; providing educative advice on rehabilitation for patients with burn injuries [57]. Nurse-led burn clinics and services also provide healthcare (e.g., ability to prescribe optimal wound management) to referrals with minor burns from the Accident and Emergency Unit [76, 77]. In addition, burn care nurses at nurse-led burn clinics have the authority and autonomy in performing burn wound management recognized by hospitals in the provision of care for patients with burn injuries based on the assessed needs of patients and caregivers.

## 3. Conclusion

Despite the recent developments in caregiving approaches for patients with burn injuries, morbidity and mortality continue to increase worldwide. Several comprehensive programs related to burn care have been implemented to enhance nurse's competency to care for patients with burn injuries in the acute care framework. In Hong Kong, burn care nurses at nurse-led clinic educate patients with burn injuries and their families/caregivers throughout the hospitalization period, discharge planning, and rehabilitative journey to ease their anxiety and promote recovery. Moreover, burn care nurses attend continuing education programs, in-service training programs, and both local and international conferences to enhance their knowledge and readiness to respond to burns injuries, as well as management and leadership in local practice with a global perspective. Nurse-led clinic and referral pathway can reduce patient hospitalization and foster better long-term rehabilitation and return home. The incentives of Hospital Authority to increase the number of nurses attending burn care training courses to enhance high quality care to patients with burn injuries. No LDI study has objectively assessed the different severity of burn depth of perform by nurses; therefore, we recommend that burn care nurses conduct a study focusing on the objective LDI assessment of diverse severity of burn depth.

## Funding

This research received funding support from the Institutional Development Grant of the Caritas Institute of Higher Education, grant number IDG220225.

## Conflict of interest

The authors declare no conflict of interest.

## Notes/thanks/other declarations

None.

## Author details

Tze-Wing Wong[1], Ka-Huen Yip[2]*, Yuk-Chiu Yip[3] and Wai-King Tsui[2]

1 Princes of Wales Hospital, Shatin, Hong Kong, China

2 Caritas Institute of Higher Education, Hong Kong, China

3 Hong Kong Metropolitan University, Hong Kong, China

*Address all correspondence to: khyip@cihe.edu.hk

## References

[1] Kelly C, Wallace D, Moulin V, Germain L, Zuccaro J, Galdyn I, et al. Surviving an extensive burn injury using advanced skin replacement technologies. Journal of Burn Care & Research. 2021;**42**:1288-1291. DOI: 10.1093/jbcr/irab146

[2] Miller SF, Bessey PQ, Schurr MJ, Browning SM, Jeng JC, Caruso DM, et al. National Burn Repository 2005: A ten-year review. Journal of Burn Care & Research. 2006;**27**:411-436. DOI: 10.1097/01.BCR.0000226260.17523.22

[3] Evers LH, Bhavsar D, Mailänder P. The biology of burn injury. Experimental Dermatology. 2010;**19**:777-783. DOI: 10.1111/j.1600-0625.2010.01105.x

[4] Tan T, Ko WS, Chan PL, Tse DA, Chiu TW. Epidemiology of paediatric burns in a tertiary Centre in Hong Kong: A 10-year review. Surgical Practice. 2021;**25**:146-151. DOI: 10.1111/1744-1633.12508

[5] Loos MHJ, Almekinders CAM, Heymans MW, de Vries A, Bakx R. Incidence and characteristics of non-accidental burns in children: A systematic review. Burns: Journal of the International Society for Burn Injuries. 2020;**46**:1243-1253. DOI: 10.1016/j.burns.2020.01.008

[6] Hemeda M, Maher A, Mabrouk A. Epidemiology of burns admitted to Ain Shams University burns unit, Cairo, Egypt. Burns: Journal of the International Society for Burn Injuries. 2003;**29**:353-358. DOI: 10.1016/s0305-4179(03)00044-5

[7] Khadim MF, Rashid A, Fogarty B, Khan K. Mortality estimates in the elderly burn patients: The Northern Ireland experience. Burns: Journal of the International Society for Burn Injuries. 2009;**35**:107-113. DOI: 10.1016/j.burns.2008.05.004

[8] Pham TN, Kramer CB, Wang J, Rivara FP, Heimbach DM, Gibran NS, et al. Epidemiology and outcomes of older adults with burn injury: An analysis of the National Burn Repository. Journal of Burn Care & Research: Official Publication of the American Burn Association. 2009;**30**:30-36. DOI: 10.1097/BCR.0b013e3181921efc

[9] Tracy LM, Singer Y, Schrale R, Gong J, Darton A, Wood F, et al. Epidemiology of burn injury in older adults: An Australian and New Zealand perspective. Scars, Burns & Healing. 2020;**6**:2059513120952336. DOI: 10.1177/2059513120952336

[10] Al-Mousawi AM, Mecott-Rivera GA, Jeschke MG, Herndon DN. Burn teams and burn centers: The importance of a comprehensive team approach to burn care. Clinics in Plastic Surgery. 2009;**36**:547-554. DOI: 10.1016/j.cps.2009.05.015

[11] Hughes A, Almeland SK, Leclerc T, Ogura T, Hayashi M, Mills JA, et al. Recommendations for burns care in mass casualty incidents: WHO emergency medical teams technical working group on burns (WHO TWGB) 2017-2020. Burns: Journal of the International Society for Burn Injuries. 2021;**47**:349-370. DOI: 10.1016/j.burns.2020.07.001

[12] Tottoli EM, Dorati R, Genta I, Chiesa E, Pisani S, Conti B. Skin wound healing process and new emerging technologies for skin wound care and regeneration. Pharmaceutics.

2020;**12**:735. DOI: 10.3390/pharmaceutics12080735

[13] Australian & New Zealand Burn Association. Emergency Management of Severe Burns Course Manual. Queensland: Australia & New Zealand Burn Association; 2006

[14] Choi EP, Chin WY, Wan EY, Lam CL. Evaluation of the internal and external responsiveness of the pressure ulcer scale for haling (PUSH) tool for assess acute and chronic wounds. Journal of Advanced Nursing. 2016;**72**:1134-1143. DOI: 10.1111/jan.12898

[15] Hospital Authority Head Office. Service Networking of Burn Service, HAHO Operations Circular No. 1/2017. Hong Kong, China: Hospital Authority; 2017

[16] ISBI Practice Guidelines Committee, Advisory Subcommittee, Steering Subcommittee. ISBI practice guidelines for burn care, part 2. Burns: Journal of the International Society for Burn Injuries. 2018;**44**:1617-1706. DOI: 10.1016/j.burns.2018.09.012

[17] Collis N, Smith G, Fenton OM. Accuracy of burn size estimation and subsequent fluid resuscitation prior to arrival at the Yorkshire regional burns unit. A three year retrospective study. Burns: Journal of the International Society for Burn Injuries. 1999;**25**:345-351. DOI: 10.1016/s0305-4179(99)00007-8

[18] Freiburg C, Igneri P, Sartorelli K, Rogers F. Effects of differences in percent total body surface area estimation on fluid resuscitation of transferred burn patients. Journal of Burn Care & Research. 2007;**28**:42-48. DOI: 10.1097/BCR.0B013E31802C88B2

[19] Hagstrom M, Wirth GA, Evans GR, Ikeda CJ. A review of emergency department fluid resuscitation of burn patients transferred to a regional, verified burn center. Annals of Plastic Surgery. 2003;**51**:173-176. DOI: 0.1097/01.SAP.0000058494.24203.99

[20] James SL, Lucchesi LR, Bisignano C, Castle CD, Dingels ZV, Fox JT, et al. Epidemiology of injuries from fire, heat and hot substances: Global, regional and national morbidity and mortality estimates from the global burden of disease 2017 study. Injury Prevention. 2020;**26**:i36-i45. DOI: 10.1136/injuryprev-2019-043299

[21] Brandt CP, Yowler CJ, Fratianne RB. Burns with multiple trauma. The American Journal of Surgery. 2002;**68**:240

[22] Hawkins A, Maclennan PA, McGwin G Jr, Cross JM, Rue LW. The impact of combined trauma and burns on patient mortality. The Journal of Trauma and Acute Care Surgery. 2005;**58**:284. DOI: 10.1097/01.ta.0000130610.19361.bd

[23] Kauvar DS, Wolf SE, Wade CE, Cancio LC, Renz EM, Holcom JB. Burns sustained in combat explosions in operations Iraqi and enduring freedom (OIF/OEF explosion burns). Burns. 2006;**32**:853. DOI: 10.1016/j.burns.2006.03.008

[24] Rosenkranz KM, Sheridan R. Management of the burned trauma patient: Balancing conflicting priorities. Burns. 2002;**28**:665. DOI: 10.1016/s0305-4179(02)00109-2

[25] Santaniello JM, Luchette FA, Esposito TJ, Gunawan H, Reed RL, Davis KA, et al. Ten year experience of burn, trauma, and combined burn/trauma injuries comparing outcomes. Journal of Trauma and Acute Care Surgery. 2004;**7**:696. DOI: 10.1097/01.ta.0000140480.50079.a8

[26] World Health Organization. Burns. 2018. Available from: https://www.who.int/news-room/fact-sheets/detail/burns [Accessed: December 8, 2022]

[27] Olszewski A, Yanes A, Stafford J, Greenhalgh DG, Palmieri TL, Sen S, et al. Development and implementation of an innovative burn nursing handbook for quality improvement. Journal of Burn Care & Research: Official Publication of the American Burn Association. 2016;**37**:20-24. DOI: 10.1097/BCR.0000000000000299

[28] Shivanpour M, Firouzkouhi M, Abdollahi Mohammad A, Naderifar M, Mohammadi M. Nurses experiences in the burn unit: A qualitative research. Iranian Journal of Nursing and Midwifery Research. 2020;**25**:232-236. DOI: 10.4103/ijnmr.IJNMR_162_19

[29] Veenema TG, editor. Disaster Nursing and Emergency Preparedness. New York: Springer Publishing Company; 2018

[30] Langan JC, Lavin R, Wolgast KA, Veenema TG. Education for developing and sustaining a health care workforce for disaster readiness. Nursing Administration Quarterly. 2017;**41**:118-127. DOI: 10.1097/NAQ.0000000000000225

[31] Loke AY, Fung OW. Nurses' competencies in disaster nursing: Implications for curriculum development and public health. International Journal of Environmental Research and Public Health. 2014;**11**:3289-3303. DOI: 10.3390/ijerph110303289

[32] Said NB, Molassiotis A, Chiang VC. Psychological preparedness for disasters among nurses with disaster field experience: An international online survey. International Journal of Disaster Risk Reduction. 2020;**46**:101533. DOI: 10.1016/j.ijdrr.2020.101533

[33] Loke AY, Guo C, Molassiotis A. Development of disaster nursing education and training programs in the past 20 years (2000-2019): A systematic review. Nurse Education Today. 2021;**99**:104809. DOI: 10.1016/j.nedt.2021.104809

[34] Najafi Ghezeljeh T, Mohammad Aliha J, Haghani H, Javadi N. Effect of education using the virtual social network on the knowledge and attitude of emergency nurses of disaster preparedness: A quasi-experiment study. Nurse Education Today. 2019;**73**:88-93. DOI: 10.1016/j.nedt.2018.12.001

[35] Lee PH, Fu B, Cai W, Chen J, Yuan Z, Zhang L, et al. The effectiveness of an online training program for improving knowledge of fire prevention and evacuation of healthcare workers: A randomized controlled trial. PLoS One. 2018;**13**:e0199747. DOI: 10.1371/journal.pone.0199747

[36] Carrougher GJ, Burton-Williams K, Gauthier K, Gloger A, Remington L, Yukon K. Burn nurse competency utilization: Report from the 2019 annual American burn association meeting. Journal of Burn Care & Research. 2020;**41**:41-47. DOI: 10.1093/jbcr/irz188

[37] NHS Commissioning Board. D06/S/a NHS Standard Contract for Specialised Burns Care (All ages). The NHS England. 2013. Available from: https://www.england.nhs.uk/wp-content/uploads/2014/04/d06-spec-burn-care-0414.pdf

[38] National Network for Burn Care. National Burn Care Standards. The NHS England. 2013. Available from: https://www.britishburnassociation.org/

wpcontent/uploads/2017/06/National_Burn_Care_Standards_2013.pdf

[39] Sheridan R. Burns: A Practical Approach to Immediate Treatment and Long-Term Care. London: Manson; 2012

[40] Butler DP. The 21st century burn care team. Burns: Journal of the International Society for Burn Injuries. 2013;**39**:375-379. DOI: 10.1016/j.burns.2013.01.004

[41] Maxson PM, Dozois EJ, Holubar SD, Wrobleski DM, Dube JAO, Klipfel JM, et al. Enhancing nurse and physician collaboration in clinical decision making through high-Fidelity interdisciplinary simulation training. In: Mayo Clinic Proceedings. Amsterdam: Elsevier; 2011. pp. 31-36

[42] George KL, Quatrara B. Interprofessional simulations promote knowledge retention and enhance perceptions of teamwork skills in a surgical-trauma-burn intensive care unit setting. Dimensions of Critical Care Nursing. 2018;**37**:144-155. DOI: 10.1097/DCC.0000000000000301

[43] Oliveira-Kumakura ARDS, Silva JLG, Gonçalves N. From theory to simulation to teach care for burn victims: Case report. Escola Anna Nery. 2018;**22**:e20170391. DOI: 10.1590/2177-9465-EAN-2017-0391

[44] Sadideen H, Wilson D, Moiemen N, Kneebone R. Using "the burns suite" as a novel high fidelity simulation tool for interprofessional and teamwork training. Journal of Burn Care & Research: Official Publication of the American Burn Association. 2016;**37**:235-242. DOI: 10.1097/BCR.0000000000000262

[45] Hong Kong College of Surgical Nursing. Course: Surgical Nursing Training (Part A) OnlineLecture Series [Internet]. 2022. Available from: https://www.hkcsn.org.hk/courses [Accessed: November 30, 2022]

[46] American Burn Association. Annual Meeting [Internet]. 2022. Available from: https://ameriburn.org/education/annual-meeting/ [Accessed: November 30, 2022]

[47] Ignatavicius D, Chung CE. Professional development for nursing faculty: Assessing transfer of learning into practice. Teaching and Learning in Nursing. 2016;**11**:138-142. DOI: 10.1016/j.teln.2016.05.005

[48] Norman G, Christie J, Liu Z, Westby MJ, Jefferies JM, Hudson T, et al. Antiseptics for burns. Cochrane Database of Systematic Reviews. 2019;**7**:CD011821. DOI: 10.1002/14651858.CD011821.pub2

[49] Wasiak J, Cleland H, Campbell F, Spinks A. Dressings for superficial and partial thickness burns. Cochrane Database of Systematic Reviews. 2013;**2013**:CD002106. DOI: 10.1002/14651858.CD002106.pub4

[50] Niazi ZB, Essex TJ, Papini R, Scott D, McLean NR, Black MJ. New laser Doppler scanner, a valuable adjunct in burn depth assessment. Burns: Journal of the International Society for Burn Injuries. 1993;**19**:485-489. DOI: 10.1016/0305-4179(93)90004-r

[51] Gill P. The critical evaluation of laser Doppler imaging in determining burn depth. International Journal of Burns and Trauma. 2013;**3**:72-77

[52] Hop MJ, Hiddingh J, Stekelenburg C, Kuipers HC, Middelkoop E, Nieuwenhuis MK, et al. LDI study group. Cost-effectiveness of laser Doppler imaging in burn care in the Netherlands. BMC Surgery. 2013;**13**:2. DOI: 10.1186/1471-2482-13-2

[53] Jan SN, Khan FA, Bashir MM, Nasir M, Ansari HH, Shami HB, et al. Comparison of laser doppler imaging (LDI) and clinical assessment in differentiating between superficial and deep partial thickness burn wounds. Burns: Journal of the International Society for Burn Injuries. 2018;**44**:405-413. DOI: 10.1016/j.burns.2017.08.020

[54] Pape SA, Baker RD, Wilson D, Hoeksema H, Jeng JC, Spence RJ, et al. Burn wound healing time assessed by laser Doppler imaging (LDI). Part 1: Derivation of a dedicated colour code for image interpretation. Burns: Journal of the International Society for Burn Injuries. 2012;**38**:187-194. DOI: 10.1016/j.burns.2010.11.009

[55] Khatib M, Jabir S, Fitzgerald O'Connor E, Philp B. A systematic review of the evolution of laser Doppler techniques in burn depth assessment. Plastic Surgery International. 2014;**2014**:621792. DOI: 10.1155/2014/621792

[56] Shin JY, Yi HS. Diagnostic accuracy of laser Doppler imaging in burn depth assessment: Systematic review and meta-analysis. Burns: Journal of the International Society for Burn Injuries. 2016;**42**:1369-1376. DOI: 10.1016/j.burns.2016.03.012

[57] Herndon DN. Total Burn Care. 5th ed. London: W.B. Saunders Company; 2018

[58] Clayton MC, Solem LD. No ice, no butter: Advice on management of burns for primary care physicians. Postgraduate Medicine. 1995;**97**:151-165. DOI: 10.1080/00325481.1995

[59] Mertens DM, Jenkins ME, Warden GD. Outpatient burn management. The Nursing clinics of North America. 1997;**32**:343-364

[60] Peate WF. Outpatient management of burns. American Family Physician. 1992;**45**:1321-1330

[61] Cancio LC. Topical antimicrobial agents for burn wound care: History and current status. Surgical Infections. 2021;**22**:3-11. DOI: 10.1089/sur.2020.368

[62] Stoica AE, Chircov C, Grumezescu AM. Naomaterials for wound dressings: An up-to-date overview. Molecules. 2020;**25**:2699. DOI: 10.3390/molecules25112699

[63] Yoshino Y, Ohtsuka M, Kawaguchi M, Sakai K, Hashimoto A, Hayashi M, et al. Wound/burn guidelines committee. The wound/burn guidelines–6: Guidelines for the management of burns. The. Journal of Dermatology. 2016;**43**:989-1010. DOI: 10.1111/1346-8138.13288

[64] Severing AL, Rembe JD, Koester V, Stuermer EK. Safety and efficacy profiles of different commercial sodium hypochlorite/hypochlorous acid solutions (NaClO/HClO): Antimicrobial efficacy, cytotoxic impact and physicochemical parameters in vitro. The Journal of Antimicrobial Chemotherapy. 2019;**74**:365-372. DOI: 10.1093/jac/dky432

[65] Finnerty CC, Jeschke MG, Branski LK, Barret JP, Dziewulski P, Herndon DN. Hypertrophic scarring: The greatest unmet challenge after burn injury. The Lancet. 2016;**388**:1427-1436. DOI: 10.1016/S0140-6736(16)31406-4

[66] Knighton J. Nursing management of the burn patient. In: Jeschike MG, Kamolz LP, Sjöberg F, Wolf SE, editors. Handbook of Burns. Vol. 1. New York: Springer; 2020. pp. 347-384

[67] Greenwood JE, Wagstaff MJ, Rooke M, Caplash Y. Reconstruction of extensive calvarial exposure after

major burn injury in 2 stages using a biodegradable polyurethane matrix. Eplasty. 2016;**16**:e17

[68] Larson KW, Austin CL, Thompson SJ. Treatment of a full-thickness burn injury with NovoSorb biodegradable temporizing matrix and RECELL autologous skin cell suspension: A case series. Journal of Burn Care & Research: Official Publication of the American Burn Association. 2020;**41**:215-219. DOI: 10.1093/jbcr/irz179

[69] Lo CH, Brown JN, Dantzer EJG, Maitz PKM, Vandervord JG, Wagstaff MJD, et al. Wound healing and dermal regeneration in severe burn patients treated with NovoSorb® biodegradable Temporising matrix: A prospective clinical study. Burns: Journal of the International Society for Burn Injuries. 2022;**48**:529-538. DOI: 10.1016/j.burns.2021.07.014

[70] Greenwood JE, Schmitt BJ, Wagstaff MJ. Experience with a synthetic bilayerbiodegradable temporising matrix in significant burn injury. Burns Open. 2018;**2**:17-34. DOI: 10.1016/j.burnso.2017.08.001

[71] Widjaja W, Tan J, Maitz PKM. Efficacy of dermal substitute on deep dermal to full thickness burn injury: A systematic review. ANZ Journal of Surgery. 2017;**87**:446-452. DOI: 10.1111/ans.13920

[72] Yiğitbaş H, Yavuz E, Beken Özdemir E, Onen O, Pençe HH, Meriç S, et al. Our experience with dermal substitute Nevelia® in the treatment of severely burned patients. Ulusal Travma ve Acil Cerrahi Dergisi. 2019;**25**:520-526. DOI: 10.14744/tjtes.2019.24358

[73] Heimbach DM, Warden GD, Luterman A, Jordan MH, Ozobia N, Ryan CM, et al. Multicenter postapproval clinical trial of Integra® dermal regeneration template for burn treatment. The Journal of Burn Care & Rehabilitation. 2003;**24**:42-48. DOI: 10.1097/00004630-200301000-00009

[74] Dill V, Mörgelin M. Biological dermal templates with native collagen scaffolds provide guiding ridges for invading cells and may promote structured dermal wound healing. International Wound Journal. 2020;**17**:618-630. DOI: 10.1111/iwj.13314

[75] Atiyeh BS. Nonsurgical management of hypertrophic scars: Evidence-based therapies, standard practices, and emerging methods. Aesthetic Plastic Surgery. 2007;**31**:468-492. DOI: 10.1007/s00266-006-0253-y

[76] Edwards J. The challenge of developing a nurse-led burns clinic. WOUNDS UK. 2007;**3**:44-50

[77] Hatchett R. The emergence of the modern nurse-led clinic. In: Nurse-Led Clinics. Oxfordshire: Routledge; 2013. pp. 15-40

Chapter 9

# Physiological and Physical Effects of Sleep Disorder among Shift Work Nurses

*Razzagh Rahimpoor*

## Abstract

Poor sleep quality as one of the mental problems caused by shift working can lead to psychological disorders (i.e., depression; adult attention deficit; memory, cognitive, and performance deficit; reduced job satisfaction, quality of life, and sex drive; and mood change) and physiological disorders (immune system, obesity, cardiovascular risks, hormone imbalance, fertility, and aging). The main scope of the proposed chapter is to describe the various dimensions of psychological and physiological disorders caused by poor sleep quality among shift-working nurses. Also, educational programs will be described for early detection of physiological and psychological symptoms of poor-quality sleep and improvement of sleep quality among shift-working nurses.

**Keywords:** nurses, sleep disorders, night shift work, circadian rhythm, health status

## 1. Introduction

Sleep plays a vital role in brain function and systemic physiology across many body systems [1]. Sleep is controlled by the Supra Chiasmatic Nucleus (SCN) of the hypothalamus, the endogenous clock that regulates the production of melatonin, a hormone that induces sleep [2]. Sleep plays an essential role in brain function, and also, the quantity and quality of sleep affect the systemic physiology of the body, including appetite regulation, metabolism, and the function of the immune, cardiovascular, and hormonal systems [3, 4].

Normal sound sleep is defined by adequate duration, good quality, suitable timing and arrangements, and no sleep disturbances [5]. Sleep is one of the most important parameters in night cycles, which plays a key role in restoring physical and emotional strength [6]. Around a third of human life is spent on sleep, and more than thirty percent of the world's people suffer from sleep disruptions because of mental-psychological illness, physical diseases, night work, second employment, and so on. The health care system is one of the most important areas of sustainable human health development where nurses are the main occupational group in the therapeutic system. Nurses usually make up forty percent of the hospital staff, and more than half of the total personnel costs are allocated to them [7–9]. At night, employees of public service-providing areas are working, so that 36.9% of the hospital staff are night-working individuals, and they are often nurses [10].


IntechOpen

The results of decades of research have indicated that sleep disruption or insomnia is a widespread problem among people bearing depression; most of them complain of difficulty in starting and maintaining sleep, waking up early in the morning, difficulty in returning to sleep, and insufficient quality of sleep [11–13]. Problems with sleep are widely prevalent and include deficits in quantity and quality of sleep; sleep problems that impact the continuity of sleep are collectively referred to as sleep disruptions [1]. Sleep deprivation is used to refer to acute total sleep deprivation (typically short periods of wakefulness (<72 h) accompanied by a nearly complete loss (>90%) of both non-Rapid Eye Movement [REM] sleep and REM sleep). The non-REM sleep is often caused by occupational demands as experienced by emergency workers, shift workers, and medicine physicians on 36–48 h work shifts by clinical conditions or in military personnel due to insomnia [14].

Sleep disorders tend to occur in one of three ways: inability to obtain a sufficient amount or quality of sleep (called sleep deprivation), unable to maintain sleep durability (difficulty maintaining sleep, called disrupted sleep or sleep fragmentation, and middle insomnia), and what events happen during sleep (for example, restless legs syndrome or sleep apnea) [1, 3].

Sleepiness is the desire or inclination to sleep, whereas fatigue is the lack of desire or disinclination to continue performing the task at hand [15]. Numerous factors contribute to sleep disruption, ranging from lifestyle and environmental factors to sleep disorders and other medical conditions. Sleep disruptions have substantial adverse short- and long-term health consequences [1]. Several studies have shown that the mortality rate in people with a sleep time of fewer than 3.5 h and more than 8.5 h is higher than in those people with a sleep duration of 7 h a day [10, 16, 17].

Physiological systems that follow circadian rhythms like the sleep-wake cycle, hormone secretions, and core body temperature are influenced by signals from the environment especially light [18]. Altered circadian rhythm results in physiological and psychological variables [19, 20]. Shift work results in a conflict between days-oriented circadian physiology and the requirement for work and sleeps at the wrong biological time of day. Internally driven circadian biological clocks regulate the periods of sleepiness and wakefulness [20]. Sleep deprivation affects the ability of health workers who are involved in a multitude of life-saving tasks that need more attention and concentration. Quality of sleep is compromised in those who are frequently involved in extended working hours and shift work, which is found to be more common among nurses [21].

## 2. Shift work

Rotating and scheduling are the main characteristics of shift work, and nurses are largely locked into schedules that provide 24-h care and include night-shift work [22, 23]. The "shift workers are creators and victims at the same time" of this new work organization [24].

Nursing professionals being one of the most vulnerable populations with chronic work stress due to the high degree of relationship between nurses and patients and the strong emotional involvement that this requires [25]. Nursing is inherently a stressful profession requiring comparatively high levels of physical and mental activity [26]. There are several stressful situations in the nursing profession that can cause problems, including dissatisfaction, low efficiency, and retirement. These situations result in physical and mental health issues that irreversibly damage the nursing system [27]. Previous studies have shown that high stress among nurses has affected their quality of professional life [28, 29].

Continuous and extended work in close proximity to patients, numerous and strenuous work shifts, poor levels of independence, dissatisfaction with occupational responsibilities, and unprepared to deal with emotional events are some specificities innate to the work of nursing technicians and nursing assistants that make them more prone to developing sleep disorders [30]. Shift work disorder is distinguished as a sleep disorder specified by insomnia in a person's daily scheme [31]. Working on the night shift has been inverse to human nature and induces various disturbances in the night-time rhythm (circadian rhythm: biological clock) and other undesirable health effects, such as digestive disorders, cardiovascular disorders, and reproductive system disorders, and raises accident rates and decreases efficacy among employees [32, 33]. The nature of the nursing job and their occupational stress, along with the harmful physical factors, are the reason for sleep disorders and drowsiness during the daytime [34].

In addition to adverse health consequences and diminished quality of life at the individual level, shift work disorder incurs significant costs to employers through diminished workplace performance and increased accidents and errors [35]. Recent scientific findings have provided insight into individual differences in tolerance for shift work and expanded cure options for persons with shift-related work disorders. At the same time, attempts to diminish the burden of shift work among employees are still at an early stage. Despite the insufficient data, from an organizational standpoint, reducing the costs related to shift work has the potential to generate significant financial benefits [35]. Furthermore, occupational demands are frequent causes of insufficient sleep and may elevate the risk of accidents at work [36].

Cognitive impairment leads to fatigability and a decline in attention and efficiency in the workplace, which puts nurses' health and patients' health at risk. Cognitive performance is impaired among shift-working nurses, due to poor sleep quality and decreased alertness during the wake state [20]. Night work worsens the well-being of the employee and accelerates the accumulation of fatigue, which is the cause of lower quality and efficiency of work and numerous absences of the employee. Working at the night shift is attended by excessive stress, which makes it very hard to rest and sleep adequately [37, 38]. The result of this is the occurrence of many diseases, including diabetes, hypertension, ischemic heart disease, neurosis, anxiety disorders, and depression, which subsequently lead to various sick leaves, occupational burnout, and incompatibility with the environment and with families [39].

Working at night disrupts all of the physiological processes of the body, as well as causes an increase in the stress hormones adrenaline and cortisol, which are the main representatives of glucocorticoid hormones. Sleep deprivation raises the level of cortisol in blood serum, which subsequently arranges the body to a constant state of readiness. Because of this, higher levels of cortisol hormone cannot go back to normal levels in spite of sleeping at night [38]. It is thought that a long-term adaptation to night-shift work is extremely restricted or even inevitable [40].

## 3. Psychological disorders

Nurses work rotating shifts and extended hours, which can change the circadian rhythm, occasionally leading to abuse of caffeine and benzodiazepines and nurses needing to use their days off and free time to recover from lost sleep hours. On the other hand, the consequences that arise from nurse burnout are numerous, such as absenteeism; lack of motivation; concentration difficulty; poor organization; increased errors; decreased patient safety; lack of energy; and feelings of frustration, anxiety, and depression; and insomnia. This scenario leads to poor sleep quality, which plays a critical role in emotional regulation and mental well-being, creating a cyclical issue underlying nursing work [25, 41].

One of the responsibilities of a nurse is prescribing the right drug on time to the right patient by the correct route. Therefore, it is obligatory that nurses clarify obscure orders; have the requisite knowledge and strength of character to question orders that are inappropriate; doubly and triply verify the medicinal product, dosage, and identity of the patient; administer the drug at the correct time and through the right route; and carefully monitor the patient [42]. Administering drugs is part of everyday nursing practice. Patient safety is a key concern in today's healthcare delivery systems. Errors in medication administration can pose a threat to patient outcomes and patient safety [43].

Research conducted among night-shift residents' and nurses reported that poor concentration hindered their efficient, decision-making capacity and also caused increased error rates. Better cognitive ability was reported among nurses who had never been exposed to shifting work compared to those who had been exposed to sleep deprivation, altered circadian rhythm, and extended shift work duration [11, 44]. Chronic fatigue, emotional exhaustion, cognitive anxiety, and worse sleep quality are more common among shift-work nurses than other nurses, and it is associated with the duration of their work shift. In other words, the increase in days of rest for 12-h shift nurses does not seem to be sufficient to neutralize the accumulation of adverse effects during extended workdays [45]. Due to the high incidence of medical mistakes and significant gaps in healthcare quality (medication errors and patient deaths), patient safety is a key concern of today's healthcare delivery systems, and medication administration errors are frequently used as an indicator of patient safety. Several studies have shown that failure to obtain adequate sleep is an important contributor to medical errors, and sleep deprivation can make many healthcare workers, including nurses, more susceptible to irritation and anger toward those they care about. It often causes feelings of guilt, depression, and anxiety and more sleep disorders. Difficulty in sleeping significantly increases the risk of depression even in someone who hasn't had a history of depression before [32].

Several studies have investigated the effect of sleep loss on the development of these neurons [46]. Disruption of sleep for one night appears to have little effect on the rate of cell production, but chronic sleep restriction or disruption of sleep has cumulative effects that lead to a reduction of neuronal development [47, 48]. Additionally, sleep restriction interferes with the normal increase in neurogenesis that occurs with hippocampus-dependent learning tasks (e.g., spatial learning) [49]. It is hypothesized that decreases in cell production are related to a decrease in REM sleep commonly seen in total sleep deprivation and sleep restriction [50].

Partial sleep deprivation reduces response inhibition during the night shift and frontal-lobe vulnerability. Working memory and episodic memory are related to temporal-lobe function, and therefore, relative sleep deprivation has detrimental effects on the psychiatric health of nurses on duty, which is responsible for impaired memory, concentration, and thinking ability [20]. A medical error is defined as a situation when a healthcare professional chooses the wrong method of care or a situation in which the healthcare professional selects the right method of care but performs it incorrectly; so medical errors are frequently described as human errors in the healthcare system [51, 52]. Shift work leads to experiencing circadian disturbance, particularly working overnight shifts or rotating shifts; also, shift work schedules increase the risk of accidents and injuries [53]. Working during the evening or night can lead to aggravating fatigue in employees because the circadian cycle is disrupted, and on the other hand, fatigue can increase the rate of human errors as a part of medical errors [54]. The cognitive deficits associated with total sleep deprivation have been well described by many studies.

Various studies have continually shown a deleterious effect of total sleep deprivation on vigilant attention. Other cognitive domains aside from attention have also been found to deteriorate with total sleep deprivation. These include spatial working memory, verbal memory, constructive thinking, and cognitive throughput [55–58]. Total sleep deprivation can result in task perseveration with reduced creative thinking and an inability to perceive the likelihood of making errors [57, 59]. Results of previous studies revealed that wrong time and wrong rate were the most frequent medication errors committed by nurses. These errors may be due to either oral or written miscommunication, name confusion, similar or misleading container labeling, or performance or knowledge deficits [15, 60]. People's instability starts when the biological mechanisms affecting the sleep initiation process interfere with cognitive functions. This makes cognitive functions more variable and dependent more and more on intentional efforts to stay awake. The aftereffects of state instability are manifested by increasingly frequent errors of commission (responding when not required) and errors of omission (not responding when it is required) [50, 61].

The most frequent complaints among nurses have been reported as insufficient sleep, short sleep duration, and insomnia [62]. External, environmental, and social factors may also act as predisposing factors for poor sleep. During periods of stressful events and changes in routine, sleep quality may be negatively affected [63]. Sleep plays a fundamental role in learning, memory consolidation, and motor learning, as well as in the immune system and cardiovascular and liver metabolism [25]. Deficits in attention, learning & memory, sensory perception, emotional reactivity, and higher-order cognitive processes, such as executive function and decision-making, have all been documented following sleep disruption in humans [14].

Short-term consequences of sleep disruption include increased stress responsivity; somatic problems; reduced quality of life; emotional distress; mood disorders and other mental health problems; cognition, memory, and performance deficits; and behavior problems in otherwise healthy individuals [1].

Stress and emotional tension from exhausting working conditions can cause burnout syndrome. Burnout is an emotional disorder with symptoms such as stress, fatigue, and physical exhaustion resulting from very stressful work associated with a high degree of responsibility or competitiveness [64]. Burnout groups also show greater sleep fragmentation, lower sleep efficiency, less slow wave and Rapid Eye Movement sleep, lower delta power density in non-REM sleep, and finally lower subjective sleep quality [65].

Burnout can have severe impacts on patients and healthcare professionals. This not only leads to negative mental and physical health outcomes, absenteeism, poor morale, and lack of incentive among personnel but also results in a decline in the quality of care delivered by the affected personnel, resulting in inferior consequences for patients [66].

Inadequate sleep or circadian changes can reduce mental performance and cognitive function, decrease levels of concentration and attention, slow down complex coordination, increase the risk of accidents, increase psychiatric morbidity, impair the cardiovascular autonomous response system, and also increase physical fatigue [67, 68]. Sleep anxiety can also mediate between depressive symptoms and sleep disorders. Sleep anxiety can be defined as a 24-h phenomenon originating from worries created by insufficient and uncontrollable sleep. Another noteworthy finding is that emotional exhaustion and sleep anxiety have successively caused the association between sleep disorders and depressive symptoms [44, 69]. Previous studies confirm that there is a significant relationship between low earnings and stress in clinical workplaces and the rate of medication errors.

Patient safety outcomes, including medication errors, have been related to occupational burnout in nurses, which is related to staff shortage, unfavourability of nurse-physician relations, and further work-life factors [43, 70].

Emotional exhaustion, job dissatisfaction, and depersonalization are significant factors that influence sleep disorders. Emotional exhaustion, which causes burnout, significantly affects the occurrence of sleep problems. Exhaustion can make work at night more tiring, while the body's ability to regenerate worsens, which may directly cause health problems [38]. Emotional exhaustion is an enduring state of physical and emotional depletion that is caused by personal demands, excessive work, and continuous stress [71]. Clearly, providing services or care, like nursing, can be a very challenging profession, and of course, emotional exhaustion is a usual response to this job overload [72]. Emotional exhaustion is a stress-related and social problem, whereas depression is a pervasive and individual problem [73]. Emotional exhaustion can be an important mediator in the relationship between sleep disturbance and depressive symptoms. Empirical studies have shown that sleep disturbance leads to increased emotional exhaustion. Emotional exhaustion represents the basic individual stress dimension of burnout, which is defined as a psychological state resulting from prolonged emotional or psychological stress on the job [70].

Nurses also typically travail from high workloads and face problems balancing work and family life. These personal workplace conflicts lead to the formation of occupational stress and burnout. In addition, the aftereffects caused by the prevalence of burnout among nurses are multiple, including lack of motivation; reduction in work performance and communication between co-workers; increased absenteeism; grown errors; deficient organization; loss of energy; reduction in patient safety; feelings of frustration, depression, and anxiety; and insomnia [73]. Several studies show that sleep pattern disorders, daytime sleepiness, and burnout are more common among shift-working nurses with 12-hr shifts or more and discontinuous or badly organized shifts than other nurses. These variables are most influenced by the fixed night shift and the rotating shift [25, 74].

Sleep deprivation raises your risk of depression, even for someone without a history of depression. Depression is a syndrome with multiple symptoms, in particular changes in one's behavior (isolation), mood (guilt and sadness), thinking and perception patterns (less focus and lower self-respect), physical complaints (sex, sleep, and hunger), and a high potential of suicide [75]. Previous studies reported significant correlation between sleep parameters and sleep quality, as well as daytime impairment [31, 76]. Several studies have demonstrated that sleep disturbance leads to symptoms of worry, which later develop into depressive symptoms and mood disorders [77, 78]. Generally, the self-reported mood is also affected by sleep deprivation. In the majority of sleep deprivation studies, there is an increase in negative mood states, with reports of fatigue and confusion as well as reduced energy and enthusiasm. Sleep restriction also affects mood [79] and sociability and has been found to exacerbate psychosomatic symptoms, including feelings of muscular pain, nausea, headache, and generalized body pain. As such, sleep restriction may degrade long-term well-being [80].

The impact of sleep disturbance on depressive symptoms has been strongly mediated by emotional exhaustion. Furthermore, sleep disorders were related to sustaining and emotional exhaustion [81, 82]. The increase in sleep disorders has been sequentially associated with increased emotional burnout and sleep-related anxiety, leading to elevated depressive symptoms. Nurses who rotated between day and night shifts were found to have more health complaints and were less satisfied with their working hours than their colleagues who worked 8-h shifts. The positive correlation between depression and the frequency of medication errors, in a way, indicates the increase of medication errors with the increase in depression [15]. These symptoms are often underestimated by professionals, who self-medicate instead of asking for help in medical or psychological consultation. Furthermore, it has a strong impact on the quality of care [83].

To increase productivity at work, a minimally stressful work environment is necessary. To deal with job stress, temperament control, intervention with control of depressive symptoms and mood, and good sleep quality of a worker, particularly for female nurses, might create an improved and more efficient work environment [84]. Female physicians, like nurses, are at risk of increased occupational stress. An increased workload can lead to severe psychological problems, such as sleep disorders and depression among female doctors, and subsequently affect their occupational and personal lives [85]. In general, shift work can lead to problems in the personal and professional lives of female workers due to the need to work at unusual hours and increased physical activity at work. As a result, woman shift workers have a higher risk of stroke than other workers [86].

## 4. Physical disorders

The tendency to sleep is regulated by the interaction between a "homeostatic pressure" to sleep and a "circadian alerting signal" that encourages wakefulness. The homeostatic pressure for sleep increases with each hour of wakefulness and dissipates with sleep. Also, the circadian alerting signal is controlled mainly in the suprachiasmatic nucleus of the anterior hypothalamus. This intrinsic coordinator of the circadian rhythm lasts approximately 24.2 h, which regulates not only sleep and wakefulness but also variable physiological functions such as blood pressure, body temperature, and hormone secretion (cortisol and melatonin) [35].

The natural light-darkness cycle is the is the strongest controller of the circadian rhythm. After light waves enter the eye (or through closed eyelids), photic stimuli are transmitted to the suprachiasmatic nucleus through the retinogeniculo-hypothalamic and retinohypothalamic pathways in the hypothalamus, and this suppresses the secretion of melatonin from the pineal gland [87].

Following nighttime work, these two opposing processes are uncoupled, and the balance of sleep and wakefulness is disturbed. It means that working at night or artificial "day" is not compatible with low melatonin secretion and high alertness. For instance, night-shift workers often fall asleep during the daytime, while at the same time, the circadian alarm signal is at its highest. Therefore, daytime sleep is fragmented and short, resulting in a lack of homeostatic sleep and low circadian excitement at night. In contrast, night work is expected to occur exactly when circadian alerting signals are weakest and sleepiness is at its strongest [35, 88].

Medical complications include increased risk for cardiovascular disease [89]; cerebrovascular events and stroke [86]; obesity [90] and metabolic disorders [91]; gastrointestinal complaints [92]; poor sexual health, including reduced fertility and problems during pregnancy [93]; and multiple forms of cancer [94]. The night shift has been associated with a higher incidence of varicose veins, appetite disturbance, and sleep disorders. Sleep deprivation has considerable consequences on people's personal life as they often postpone many personal and social activities. Inadequate sleep may jeopardize health professionals' efficacy to handle critical situations. Poor-quality sleep has been identified as a risk factor for nursing turnover [40].

The distress associated with sleep loss can create additional stress to maximize sleep, which, in turn, contributes to worsening (rather than improving) sleep disruption. Insomniacs have been shown to have increased EEG activity, abnormal hormone secretion, increased metabolic activity, and increased sympathetic nervous system activity throughout the day and night [1, 95].

The greatest change in blood pressure during the sleep period among those who work shifts is a relevant finding because blood pressure is expected to decrease during the sleep period, called a drop [96]. The lack of a drop and the severity of blood pressure is linked to sleep apnea, autonomic dysfunction, nightly overload, increase in mortality, decreased myocardial diastolic function, developing lesions in target organs like left ventricular hypertrophy, and increase in the prevalence of diabetic retinopathy and subsequent decline of glucose tolerance [97].

Sleep abnormalities affect immune function in a reciprocal manner, leading to changes in prion inflammatory cytokines, such as tumor necrosis factor, interleukins 1 and 6, and C-reactive protein. During both brief and extended arousals during sleep, increased metabolism is evidenced by increased oxygen consumption and carbon dioxide production. Chronic persistent insomnia is associated with increased secretion of adrenocorticotropic hormone and cortisol, which is present throughout a 24-h sleep-wake cycle [98–100].

Long-term consequences of sleep disruption in otherwise healthy individuals include hypertension, dyslipidemia, cardiovascular disease, weight-related issues, metabolic syndrome, and Type 2 diabetes mellitus. The increased activity of the sympathetic nervous system that is associated with sleep deprivation has substantial long-term consequences for adults and adolescents. Adults who experience sleep disruption have elevated blood pressure and an increased risk of developing hypertension. Sleep loss appears to affect energy metabolism primarily by impairing insulin sensitivity and increasing food intake. Disrupted sleep has been associated with weight gain and other weight-related issues. Sleep fragmentation can alter glucose homeostasis and decrease insulin sensitivity [1]. Shift work is also associated with a disturbed lipid profile; high triglycerides and low HDL levels are often noticed among shift workers. High triglycerides and low HDL cholesterol findings among shift workers are associated with metabolic syndrome compared to non-shift workers [91, 101].

Previous studies have documented the numerous gastrointestinal signs and disorders related to shift work for over two decades, including gastritis, dyspepsia, colitis, indigestion, peptic ulcer, appetite disorders, constipation, pain, heartburn, abdominal rumblings, inconsistent bowel movements, gastro-duodenitis, and flatulence [92, 102]. Several factors may be involved in the gastrointestinal symptoms reported among shift workers: altered circadian rhythm of stomach functions (enzyme activity, gastric secretion, and intestinal motility), drugs, types of foods eaten, psychosocial stress, and changed menstrual cycle (in women) [103].

Inflammatory markers such as C Reactive Protein (CRP) and leukocyte counts are higher in shift workers and are associated with cardiovascular diseases, atherosclerosis, stroke, and Type 2 diabetes mellitus (T2DM) [104, 105]. An increase in leukocytes is a major risk factor for ischemic stroke and a risk and prognostic indicator for cardiovascular diseases [106, 107]. Nightwork is one of the risk factors for diabetes management since A1c hemoglobin is higher in night shift workers with T2DM than in daytime workers [108]. Several studies have been published for investigating the probabilistic effects of shiftwork on the cardiovascular system without providing deterministic results [109]. Some studies have pointed out that night-shift workers have a higher relative risk of cardiovascular diseases than day workers [89, 110]. In a cohort study, it has been shown that mortality due to various causes, including cardiovascular diseases, among female rotating night-shiftwork nurses was higher than that among day-work nurses, which reflects the potentially adverse effects of rotating night shift on health and life expectancy [111]. A decade ago, the International Agency for Research on Cancer (IARC) confirmed that there was sufficient evidence to consider shift work along with circadian rhythm disturbance as a possible carcinogen (breast cancer) [112].

The occurrence and prevalence of breast cancer among woman shift workers are higher than woman daytime workers. The reason for that is the suppression of melatonin secretion due to excessive exposure to light during the night shift, and considering that the secretion of melatonin at night has an antioxidant role in the pathological and physiological functions of the body, it will ultimately lead to the susceptibility of women shift workers to breast cancer [113]. The biology and growth of normal breast tissue are controlled by genes affected by the circadian rhythm, so a disturbance in the circadian rhythm can cause breast cancer [114]. Female shift workers are at a higher risk of breast cancer compared to non-shift workers because of the disturbance of their circadian rhythms. The decrease in the secretion of cortisol and melatonin hormones causes the diffusion of a series of inflammatory indicators like as TNF-α, IL-1, and IL-2 and subsequently makes women prone to breast cancer [114, 115]. Light exposure at night among shift workers suppresses the normal release of melatonin from the pineal gland and can also stimulate the production of estrogen from the ovaries, which, in turn, can result in breast cancer [10]. Prolonged work as a shift worker is a risk factor for the occurrence of breast cancer due to circadian rhythm disturbance [116].

However, a cohort study reported that there was no significant difference in cortisol levels and any of the immune system indicators between daytime and shift workers [117]. Women are more susceptible to breast cancer if they begin shift work at a very early age and work for a long time period [118].

## 5. Operational and educational suggestions

The sleep disorders cause burnout in nurses who work shifts. This science can be used to develop strategies to prevent sleep disorders and burnout in nurses, which will also better the quality of nursing services. Identifying the key factors affecting nurse burnout can play an important role in countering this destructive phenomenon by carrying out targeted treatment actions. An efficient system of monitoring shift working schedules should be set up to decrease the occurrence and prevalence of burnout and sleep disturbances. Monitoring the statistic of night shifts, forbidding nurses from working the day after the night shift, and controlling the long adequate rest breaks all can be effective in reducing the adverse effects of night work as the major reason for sleep disorders and insomnia among shiftwork nurses [38].

In many cases, it is impossible to change the work team's organization; thus, it is necessary for these professionals to adopt measures to reduce variations in the sleep-watch rhythm, using a system of daytime naps and adjusting their personal and family rhythms to their varying work schedules and days of payment. The relationship between sleep and burnout must be taken into account to improve nurses' working conditions. Developing tunicity strategies that limit alternate in circadian rhythm and improve sleep quality can be positive [25]. The distinction between scheduled and unscheduled time worked (time that is planned in advance versus time that is unanticipated) may be more important than the actual number of work hours [15].

Shift work schedules, choosing proper nurses for shift work, and how they remedy them are main factors in the management of shift worker issues. A half-hour nap helps to effectively reduce stress levels of nurses, which allows them to return home safely at the end of their shift with less sleepiness. Making proper work schedule policies among nightshift-working nurses and their implementation can provide better healthcare to the patients and also give better sleep quality and a healthy working environment to nurses [119].

An organized ergonomic turnaround can be less detrimental to the health of nurses and more beneficial for healthcare providers. A 2 × 12 rotation (day-night) had fewer sleep disorders, and the duration of sleep was more balanced and less segmented than in the rotation of 3 × 8 (AM–PM–AM). In addition, it appears that a clockwise rotation 2 × 12 provides better recovery, in spite of 50% increase in the turnaround time. A night shift in the weekly schedule does not change the circadian rhythm and nature of cortisol level of the nurses. Sleep disturbances are especially reported among nurses in morning shifts with a 3 × 8 turnaround pattern. Shift rotation pattern, if it coincides with travel time, causes the deprivation of needed rest and sleep. In the case of an early-phase rotation (afternoon, morning, night, rest, rest, rest), difficulties related to tiredness and anxiety are linked to the fear of waking up in time the next morning [120].

Using warmer lights during night shifts can be of significant help in hospital work environments, as white light can play a key role to improve sleep quality. Furthermore, if possible, the fixed night shift should be eliminated due to its adverse effects on circadian rhythm [25]. Exposure to daylight at least 3 h a day was found to cause less stress and higher satisfaction at work. Daylight exposure has a curative effect on burnout parameters because there are a lot of studies reporting this effect of daylight on mood disorders [121].

Insomnia can be treated pharmacologically; melatonin can help in the facilitation of normalizing the aberrant circadian rhythm. Benzodiazepine receptor agonist response is good among several insomniac patients, and remission rates are very low. The National Institute for Occupational Safety and Health (NIOSH) guides workers on how to cope with stressful work-related situations and manage their daily healthy physical and mental health [119, 122].

Related mental health promotion services, such as mind-based intervention and cognitive control strategies, can be useful for improving the sleep and mental health of nurses during their work [44]. According to the principles of occupational health, proper sleep as an important category should be included in the plans to improve the workplace. Screening for sleep disorders can be utilized to triage nurses to an acceptable level of treatment based on risk (for example, clinical assessment or public health education). In this regard, health services for night-shift workers should be provided by the employer during night-shift hours. This can help healthcare providers correctly diagnose the occurrence of shift-work disorders. Treatments that focus on increasing circadian adaptation, reducing sleepiness, and improving sleep can improve the quality of life in shiftwork disorder patients. Clinicians are strongly advised to incorporate family and social support to maximize patient adherence [35].

Disturbance in the circadian rhythm can lead to insufficient sleep and subsequently to cognitive impairment and poor work performance, and to overcome it, good social support and providing a supportive work environment can be used. Preventive acts to minimize psychosocial stress at workplaces like social support, family support, and providing a favorable work environment can reduce sleep problems and also increase worker efficiency within working hours. Stress management training and techniques can help cope with sleep disturbance in certain professions such as nursing. This training can last longer and be beneficial for one's future professional career life. Controlling self-temperament and a cooperative environment among employers, employees, and colleagues can help to decrease sleep disturbance and can increase the work performance and life quality of workers. Switching night work and rotational work can improve sleep disturbances, compared to sticking to the same shift schedule. Blood pressure control and napping can also play an important role in the management of hypertension related to shift work.

## Author details

Razzagh Rahimpoor
Faculty of Health, Department of Occupational Health Engineering, Student Research Committee, Larestan University of Medical Sciences, Iran

*Address all correspondence to: razzaghrahimpoor@yahoo.com

## References

[1] Medic G, Wille M, Hemels ME. Short- and long-term health consequences of sleep disruption. Nature and Science of Sleep. 2017;**9**:151

[2] Gillette MU, Tischkau SA. Suprachiasmatic nucleus: The brain's circadian clock. Recent Progress in Hormone Research. 1999;**54**:33-58; discussion 58-39

[3] Sleep M. Institute of Medicine Committee. Research: The National Academies Collection: Reports funded by National Institutes of Health. In: Colten HR, Altevogt BM, editors. Sleep Disorders and Sleep Deprivation: An Unmet Public Health Problem. Washington (DC): National Academies Press (US); 2006

[4] CC Panel, Watson NF, Badr MS, Belenky G, Bliwise DL, Buxton OM, et al. Joint consensus statement of the american academy of sleep medicine and sleep research society on the recommended amount of sleep for a healthy adult: Methodology and discussion. Journal of Clinical Sleep Medicine. 2015;**11**:931-952

[5] Watson NF, Badr MS, Belenky G, Bliwise DL, Buxton OM, Buysse D, et al. Recommended amount of sleep for a healthy adult: A joint consensus statement of the American academy of sleep medicine and sleep research society. Journal of Clinical Sleep Medicine. 2015;**11**:591-592

[6] Bazrafshan M, Rahimpoor R, Moravveji F, Soleymaninejad N, Kavi E, Sookhak F, et al. Prevalence and effects of sleep disorders among shift work nurses. Jundishapur Journal of Chronic Disease Care. 2019;**8**:e81185

[7] Bousso RS, Poles K. Cruz DdALMd: Nursing concepts and theories. Revista da Escola de Enfermagem da USP. 2014;**48**:141-145

[8] Shoghi M, Sanjari M, Shirazi F, Heidari S, Salemi S, Mirzabeigi G. Workplace violence and abuse against nurses in hospitals in Iran. Asian Nursing Research. 2008;**2**:184-193

[9] Griffiths P, Maruotti A, Recio Saucedo A, Redfern OC, Ball JE, Briggs J, et al. Nurse staffing, nursing assistants and hospital mortality: Retrospective longitudinal cohort study. BMJ Quality & Safety. 2019;**28**:609-617

[10] Lin S-H, Liao W-C, Chen M-Y, Fan J-Y. The impact of shift work on nurses' job stress, sleep quality and self-perceived health status. Journal of Nursing Management. 2014;**22**: 604-612

[11] American Psychiatric Association A, Association AP. Diagnostic and Statistical Manual of Mental Disorders: Dsm-5. Washington, DC: American Psychiatric Association; 2013

[12] Baglioni C, Spiegelhalder K, Lombardo C, Riemann D. Sleep and emotions: A focus on insomnia. Sleep Medicine Reviews. 2010;**14**:227-238

[13] Armitage R, Hoffmann RF. Sleep eeg, depression and gender. Sleep Medicine Reviews. 2001;**5**:237-246

[14] McCoy JG, Strecker RE. The cognitive cost of sleep lost. Neurobiology of Learning and Memory. 2011;**96**:564-582

[15] Saleh AM, Awadalla NJ, El-masri YM, Sleem WF. Impacts of nurses' circadian rhythm sleep disorders, fatigue, and depression on medication administration

errors. Egyptian Journal of Chest Diseases and Tuberculosis. 2014;**63**:145-153

[16] Learthart S. Health effects of internal rotation of shifts. Nursing Standard (through 2013). 2000;**14**:34

[17] Wang X-S, Armstrong MEG, Cairns BJ, Key TJ, Travis RC. Shift work and chronic disease: The epidemiological evidence. Occupational Medicine. 2011;**61**:78-89

[18] Kuhn G. Circadian rhythm, shift work, and emergency medicine. Annals of Emergency Medicine. 2001;**37**:88-98

[19] Durmer JS, Dinges DF. Neurocognitive consequences of sleep deprivation. Seminars in Neurology. 2005;**25**:117-129

[20] Kaliyaperumal D, Elango Y, Alagesan M, Santhanakrishanan I. Effects of sleep deprivation on the cognitive performance of nurses working in shift. Journal of Clinical and Diagnostic Research: JCDR. 2017;**11**:CC01

[21] Chang YS, Wu YH, Hsu CY, Tang SH, Yang LL, Su SF. Impairment of perceptual and motor abilities at the end of a night shift is greater in nurses working fast rotating shifts. Sleep Medicine. 2011;**12**:866-869

[22] Ferri P, Guadi M, Marcheselli L, Balduzzi S, Magnani D, Di Lorenzo R. The impact of shift work on the psychological and physical health of nurses in a general hospital: A comparison between rotating night shifts and day shifts. Risk Management and Healthcare Policy. 2016;**9**:203-211

[23] Korompeli A, Muurlink O, Tzavara C, Velonakis E, Lemonidou C, Sourtzi P. Influence of shiftwork on Greek nursing personnel. Safety and Health at Work. 2014;**5**:73-79

[24] Costa G, Accattoli MP, Garbarino S, Magnavita N, Roscelli F. I disturbi del sonno in ambito lavorativo: Indirizzi di sorveglianza sanitaria, prevenzione e gestione del rischio. La Medicina del Lavoro. 2013;**104**:251-266

[25] Membrive-Jiménez MJ, Gómez-Urquiza JL, Suleiman-Martos N, Velando-Soriano A, Ariza T, De la Fuente-Solana EI, et al. Relation between burnout and sleep problems in nurses: A systematic review with meta-analysis: Healthcare. MDPI. 2022;**10**:954

[26] McNeely E. The consequences of job stress for nurses' health: Time for a check-up. Nursing Outlook. 2005;**53**:291-299

[27] Kokoroko E, Sanda MA. Effect of workload on job stress of ghanaian opd nurses: The role of coworker support. Safety and Health at Work. 2019;**10**:341-346

[28] Jafari M, Habibi Houshmand B, Maher A. Relationship of occupational stress and quality of work life with turnover intention among the nurses of public and private hospitals in selected cities of Guilan province, Iran, in 2016. Journal of Health Research in Community. 2017;**3**:12-24

[29] Lee E, Jang I. Nurses' fatigue, job stress, organizational culture, and turnover intention: A culture–work–health model. Western Journal of Nursing Research. 2020;**42**:108-116

[30] Dos Santos MA, Pereira FH, De Souza CJ, Oliveira HC, Ceolim MF, Andrechuk CRS. Sleep and professional burnout in nurses, nursing technicians, and nursing assistants during the covid-19 pandemic. The Journal of Nursing Research. 2022;**30**:e218-e218

[31] Flo E, Pallesen S, Magerøy N, Moen BE, Grønli J, Hilde Nordhus I,

et al. Shift work disorder in nurses – assessment, prevalence and related health problems. PLoS One. 2012;7:e33981

[32] Kecklund G, Axelsson J. Health consequences of shift work and insufficient sleep. BMJ. 2016;**355**:i5210

[33] Sparks K, Cooper C, Fried Y, Shirom A. The effects of hours of work on health: A meta-analytic review. In: Managerial, Occupational and Organizational Stress Research. London: Routledge; 2018. pp. 451-468

[34] Ruggiero JS, Redeker NS. Effects of napping on sleepiness and sleep-related performance deficits in night-shift workers: A systematic review. Biological Research for Nursing. 2014;**16**:134-142

[35] Wickwire EM, Geiger-Brown J, Scharf SM, Drake CL. Shift work and shift work sleep disorder: Clinical and organizational perspectives. Chest. 2017;**151**:1156-1172

[36] Mukherjee S, Patel SR, Kales SN, Ayas NT, Strohl KP, Gozal D, et al. An official American thoracic society statement: The importance of healthy sleep. Recommendations and future priorities. American Journal of Respiratory and Critical Care Medicine. 2015;**191**:1450-1458

[37] Ganesan S, Magee M, Stone JE, Mulhall MD, Collins A, Howard ME, et al. The impact of shift work on sleep, alertness and performance in healthcare workers. Scientific Reports. 2019;**9**:4635

[38] Młynarska A, Bronder M, Kolarczyk E, Manulik S, Młynarski R. Determinants of sleep disorders and occupational burnout among nurses: A cross-sectional study. International Journal of Environmental Research and Public Health. 2022;**19**:6218

[39] Hafner M, Stepanek M, Taylor J, Troxel WM, van Stolk C. Why sleep matters-the economic costs of insufficient sleep: A cross-country comparative analysis. Rand Health Q. 2017;**6**:11-11

[40] Kousloglou S, Mouzas O, Bonotis K, Roupa Z, Vasilopoulos A, Angelopoulos N. Insomnia and burnout in greek nurses. Hippokratia. 2014;**18**:150-155

[41] Yazdanshenas Ghazwin M, Kavian M, Ahmadloo M, Jarchi A, Golchin Javadi S, Latifi S, et al. The association between life satisfaction and the extent of depression, anxiety and stress among Iranian nurses: A multicenter survey. Iranian Journal of Psychiatry. 2016;**11**:120-127

[42] Aspden P, Aspden P. Preventing Medication Errors. Washington DC: National Academies Press; 2007

[43] Corrigan J. Crossing the quality chasm. Building a better delivery system. Washington DC: National Academies Press; 2005

[44] Xu S, Ouyang X, Shi X, Li Y, Chen D, Lai Y, et al. Emotional exhaustion and sleep-related worry as serial mediators between sleep disturbance and depressive symptoms in student nurses: A longitudinal analysis. Journal of Psychosomatic Research. 2020;**129**:109870

[45] Kim HS, Yeom H-A. The association between spiritual well-being and burnout in intensive care unit nurses: A descriptive study. Intensive and Critical Care Nursing. 2018;**46**:92-97

[46] Meerlo P, Mistlberger RE, Jacobs BL, Craig Heller H, McGinty D. New neurons in the adult brain: The role of sleep and consequences of sleep loss. Sleep Medicine Reviews. 2009;**13**:187-194

[47] van der Borght K, Ferrari F, Klauke K, Roman V, Havekes R, Sgoifo A, et al. Hippocampal cell proliferation across the day: Increase by running wheel activity, but no effect of sleep and wakefulness. Behavioural Brain Research. 2006;**167**:36-41

[48] Roman V, Van der Borght K, Leemburg SA, Van der Zee EA, Meerlo P. Sleep restriction by forced activity reduces hippocampal cell proliferation. Brain Research. 2005;**1065**:53-59

[49] Hairston IS, Little MTM, Scanlon MD, Barakat MT, Palmer TD, Sapolsky RM, et al. Sleep restriction suppresses neurogenesis induced by hippocampus-dependent learning. Journal of Neurophysiology. 2005;**94**:4224-4233

[50] Reynolds AC, Banks S. Total sleep deprivation, chronic sleep restriction and sleep disruption. In: Kerkhof GA, Dongen HPA, editors. Progress in Brain Research. 2010;**185**:91-103

[51] O'Sullivan E, Schofield S. Cognitive bias in clinical medicine. Journal of the Royal College of Physicians of Edinburgh. 2018;**48**:225-232

[52] Zhang J, Patel VL, Johnson TR. Medical error: Is the solution medical or cognitive? Journal of the American Medical Informatics Association. 2002;**9**:S75-S77

[53] Barger LK, Ayas NT, Cade BE, Cronin JW, Rosner B, Speizer FE, et al. Impact of extended-duration shifts on medical errors, adverse events, and attentional failures. PLoS Medicine. 2006;**3**:e487

[54] Krueger GP. A Fatigue, Performance, and Medical Error; Human Error in Medicine. Florida: CRC Press; 2018. pp. 311-326

[55] Van Dongen HP, Hursh SR. Fatigue, Performance, Errors, and Accidents; Principles and Practice of Sleep Medicine. 5th ed. Amsterdam: Elsevier Inc.; 2010. pp. 753-759

[56] Killgore WDS, Kahn-Greene ET, Lipizzi EL, Newman RA, Kamimori GH, Balkin TJ. Sleep deprivation reduces perceived emotional intelligence and constructive thinking skills. Sleep Medicine. 2008;**9**:517-526

[57] Horne J, Reyner L. Vehicle accidents related to sleep: A review. Occupational and Environmental Medicine. 1999;**56**:289-294

[58] Heuer H, Kohlisch O, Klein W. The effects of total sleep deprivation on the generation of random sequences of key-presses, numbers and nouns. The Quarterly Journal of Experimental Psychology Section A. 2005;**58**:275-307

[59] Harrison Y, Horne JA. The impact of sleep deprivation on decision making: A review. Journal of Experimental Psychology: Applied. 2000;**6**:236

[60] Leape LL, Bates DW, Cullen DJ, Cooper J, Demonaco HJ, Gallivan T, et al. Systems analysis of adverse drug events. JAMA. 1995;**274**:35-43

[61] Chua EC-P, Yeo S-C, Lee IT-G, Tan L-C, Lau P, Cai S, et al. Sustained attention performance during sleep deprivation associates with instability in behavior and physiologic measures at baseline. Sleep. 2014;**37**:27-39

[62] Silva-Costa A, Griep RH, Rotenberg L. Associations of a short sleep duration, insufficient sleep, and insomnia with self-rated health among nurses. PLoS One. 2015;**10**:e0126844

[63] Palagini L, Maria Bruno R, Gemignani A, Baglioni C, Ghiadoni L,

Riemann D. Sleep loss and hypertension: A systematic review. Current Pharmaceutical Design. 2013;**19**:2409-2419

[64] Campos JADB, Maroco J. Maslach burnout inventory-student survey: Portugal-Brazil cross-cultural adaptation. Revista de saude publica. 2012;**46**:816-824

[65] Ekstedt M, Söderström M, Åkerstedt T, Nilsson J, Søndergaard H-P, Aleksander P. Disturbed sleep and fatigue in occupational burnout. Scandinavian Journal of Work, Environment & Health. 2006;**32**:121-131

[66] Koutsimani P, Montgomery A, Georganta K. The relationship between burnout, depression, and anxiety: A systematic review and meta-analysis. Frontiers in Psychology. 2019;**10**:284

[67] Kemper KJ, Mo X, Khayat R. Are mindfulness and self-compassion associated with sleep and resilience in health professionals? The Journal of Alternative and Complementary Medicine. 2015;**21**:496-503

[68] Zhang Y, Duffy JF, De Castillero ER. Do sleep disturbances mediate the association between work-family conflict and depressive symptoms among nurses? A cross-sectional study. Journal of Psychiatric and Mental Health Nursing. 2017;**24**:620-628

[69] Jansson-Fröjmark M, Harvey AG, Lundh L-G, Norell-Clarke A, Linton SJ. Psychometric properties of an insomnia-specific measure of worry: The anxiety and preoccupation about sleep questionnaire. Cognitive Behaviour Therapy. 2011;**40**:65-76

[70] Mary Fry M, Dacey C. Factors contributing to incidents in medicine administration. Part 2. British Journal of Nursing. 2007;**16**:676-681

[71] Wright TA, Cropanzano R. Emotional exhaustion as a predictor of job performance and voluntary turnover. Journal of Applied Psychology. 1998;**83**:486

[72] Seidler A, Thinschmidt M, Deckert S, Then F, Hegewald J, Nieuwenhuijsen K, et al. The role of psychosocial working conditions on burnout and its core component emotional exhaustion—A systematic review. Journal of Occupational Medicine and Toxicology. 2014;**9**:10

[73] Adriaenssens J, Hamelink A, Bogaert PV. Predictors of occupational stress and well-being in first-line nurse managers: A cross-sectional survey study. International Journal of Nursing Studies. 2017;**73**:85-92

[74] Huang CL-C, Wu M-P, Ho C-H, Wang J-J. Risks of treated anxiety, depression, and insomnia among nurses: A nationwide longitudinal cohort study. PLoS One. 2018;**13**:e0204224

[75] Carlton G, Blegen MA. Medication-related errors: A literature review of incidence and antecedents. Annual Review of Nursing Research. 2006;**24**:19

[76] Tang NKY, Harvey AG. Correcting distorted perception of sleep in insomnia: A novel behavioural experiment? Behaviour Research and Therapy. 2004;**42**:27-39

[77] Pillai V, Drake CL. Chapter 10—Sleep and repetitive thought: The role of rumination and worry in sleep disturbance. In: Babson KA, Feldner MT, editors. Sleep and Affect. San Diego: Academic Press; 2015. pp. 201-225

[78] McGowan SK, Behar E, Luhmann M. Examining the relationship between worry and sleep: A daily process approach. Behavior Therapy. 2016;**47**: 460-473

[79] Dinges DF, Kribbs NB: Performing while Sleepy:Performing while sleepy: Effects of experimentally-induced sleepiness. In: Monk TH editor. Sleep, sleepiness and performance. New Jersey: John Wiley & Sons; 1991. pp. 97-128

[80] Haack M, Mullington JM. Sustained sleep restriction reduces emotional and physical well-being. Pain. 2005;**119**:56-64

[81] Sonnenschein M, Sorbi MJ, van Doornen LJP, Schaufeli WB, Maas CJM. Evidence that impaired sleep recovery may complicate burnout improvement independently of depressive mood. Journal of Psychosomatic Research. 2007;**62**:487-494

[82] Elfering A, Kottwitz MU, Tamcan Ö, Müller U, Mannion AF. Impaired sleep predicts onset of low back pain and burnout symptoms: Evidence from a three-wave study. Psychology, Health & Medicine. 2018;**23**:1196-1210

[83] Hsieh M-L, Li Y-M, Chang E-T, Lai H-L, Wang W-H, Wang S-C. Sleep disorder in Taiwanese nurses: A random sample survey. Nursing & Health Sciences. 2011;**13**:468-474

[84] Kikuchi Y, Nakaya M, Ikeda M, Okuzumi S, Takeda M, Nishi M. Relationship between job stress, temperament and depressive symptoms in female nurses. International Journal of Occupational Medicine and Environmental Health. 2014;**27**:426-434

[85] Győrffy Z, Dweik D, Girasek E. Workload, mental health and burnout indicators among female physicians. Human Resources for Health. 2016;**14**:12

[86] Brown DL, Feskanich D, Sánchez BN, Rexrode KM, Schernhammer ES, Lisabeth LD. Rotating night shift work and the risk of ischemic stroke. American Journal of Epidemiology. 2009;**169**:1370-1377

[87] Czeisler CA, Buxton OM. The Human Circadian Timing System and Sleep-Wake Regulation; Principles and Practice of Sleep Medicine. 5th ed. Amsterdam: Elsevier Inc.; 2010. pp. 402-419

[88] Guardiola-Lemaître B, Quera-Salva MA. Melatonin and the Regulation of Sleep and Circadian Rhythms; Principles and Practice of Sleep Medicine. Elsevier; 2011. pp. 420-430

[89] Frost P, Kolstad HA, Bonde JP. Shift work and the risk of ischemic heart disease—A systematic review of the epidemiologic evidence. Scandinavian Journal of Work, Environment & Health. 2009;**35**:163-179

[90] Caruso CC. Negative impacts of shiftwork and long work hours. Rehabilitation Nursing. 2014;**39**:16-25

[91] Karlsson B, Knutsson A, Lindahl B. Is there an association between shift work and having a metabolic syndrome? Results from a population based study of 27 485 people. Occupational and Environmental Medicine. 2001;**58**:747-752

[92] Knutsson A, Bøggild H. Gastrointestinal disorders among shift workers. Scandinavian Journal of Work, Environment & Health. 2010;**36**:85-95

[93] Mahoney MM. Shift work, jet lag, and female reproduction. International Journal of Endocrinology. 2010;**2010**:813764

[94] Jia Y, Lu Y, Wu K, Lin Q, Shen W, Zhu M, et al. Does night work increase the risk of breast cancer? A systematic review and meta-analysis of epidemiological studies. Cancer Epidemiology. 2013;**37**:197-206

[95] Meng L, Zheng Y, Hui R. The relationship of sleep duration and insomnia to risk of hypertension incidence: A meta-analysis of prospective cohort studies. Hypertension Research. 2013;**36**:985-995

[96] Nascimento JOV, Santos J, Meira KC, Pierin AMG, Souza-Talarico JN. Shift work of nursing professionals and blood pressure, burnout and common mental disorders. Revista da Escola de Enfermagem da USP. 2019;**53**:e03443

[97] Roush G, Fagard R, Salles G, Pierdomenico S, Reboldi G, Verdecchia P, et al. Prognostic impact of clinic, daytime, and nighttime systolic blood pressure in 9 cohorts of 13,843 patients with hypertension: Systematic review and meta-analysis. Journal of the American Society of Hypertension. 2014;**8**:e59

[98] Ali T, Choe J, Awab A, Wagener TL, Orr WC. Sleep, immunity and inflammation in gastrointestinal disorders. World Journal of Gastroenterology. 2013;**19**:9231-9239

[99] Hurtado-Alvarado G, Domínguez-Salazar E, Pavon L, Velázquez-Moctezuma J, Gómez-González B. Blood-brain barrier disruption induced by chronic sleep loss: Low-grade inflammation may be the link. Journal of Immunology Research. 2016;**2016**:4576012

[100] Bonnet MH, Berry RB, Arand DL. Metabolism during normal, fragmented, and recovery sleep. Journal of Applied Physiology. 1991;**71**:1112-1118

[101] Karlsson BH, Knutsson AK, Lindahl BO, Alfredsson LS. Metabolic disturbances in male workers with rotating three-shift work. Results of the wolf study. International Archives of Occupational and Environmental Health. 2003;**76**:424-430

[102] Matheson A, O'Brien L, Reid J-A. The impact of shiftwork on health: A literature review. Journal of Clinical Nursing. 2014;**23**:3309-3320

[103] Wong H, Wong MCS, Wong SYS, Lee A. The association between shift duty and abnormal eating behavior among nurses working in a major hospital: A cross-sectional study. International Journal of Nursing Studies. 2010;**47**:1021-1027

[104] Morris CJ, Purvis TE, Mistretta J, Hu K, Scheer FAJL. Circadian misalignment increases c-reactive protein and blood pressure in chronic shift workers. Journal of Biological Rhythms. 2017;**32**:154-164

[105] Puttonen S, Härmä M, Hublin C. Shift work and cardiovascular disease—Pathways from circadian stress to morbidity. Scandinavian Journal of Work, Environment & Health. 2010;**36**:96-108

[106] Lee CD, Folsom AR, Nieto FJ, Chambless LE, Shahar E, Wolfe DA. White blood cell count and incidence of coronary heart disease and ischemic stroke, and mortality from cardiovascular disease in African-American and white men and women: The atherosclerosis risk in communities study. Circulation. 2001;**103**:1357-1358

[107] Madjid M, Awan I, Willerson JT, Casscells SW. Leukocyte count and coronary heart disease. Journal of the American College of Cardiology. 2004;**44**:1945-1956

[108] Manodpitipong A, Saetung S, Nimitphong H, Siwasaranond N, Wongphan T, Sornsiriwong C, et al. Night-shift work is associated with poorer glycaemic control in patients with type 2 diabetes. Journal of Sleep Research. 2017;**26**:764-772

[109] Hublin C, Partinen M, Koskenvuo K, Silventoinen K, Koskenvuo M, Kaprio J. Shift-work and cardiovascular disease: A population-based 22-year follow-up study. European Journal of Epidemiology. 2010;**25**:315-323

[110] Ha M, Park J. Shiftwork and metabolic risk factors of cardiovascular disease. Journal of Occupational Health. 2005;**47**:89-95

[111] Gu F, Han J, Laden F, Pan A, Caporaso NE, Stampfer MJ, et al. Total and cause-specific mortality of U.S. Nurses working rotating night shifts. American Journal of Preventive Medicine. 2015;**48**:241-252

[112] Lin X, Chen W, Wei F, Ying M, Wei W, Xie X. Night-shift work increases morbidity of breast cancer and all-cause mortality: A meta-analysis of 16 prospective cohort studies. Sleep Medicine. 2015;**16**:1381-1387

[113] Leung M, Tranmer J, Hung E, Korsiak J, Day AG, Aronson KJ. Shift work, chronotype, and melatonin patterns among female hospital employees on day and night shifts. Cancer Epidemiology, Biomarkers & Prevention. 2016;**25**:830-838

[114] Blakeman V, Williams JL, Meng Q-J, Streuli CH. Circadian clocks and breast cancer. Breast Cancer Research. 2016;**18**:89

[115] Davis S, Mirick DK, Stevens RG. Night shift work, light at night, and risk of breast cancer. JNCI: Journal of the National Cancer Institute. 2001;**93**:1557-1562

[116] Schernhammer ES, Kroenke CH, Laden F, Hankinson SE. Night work and risk of breast cancer. Epidemiology. 2006;**17**:108-111

[117] Copertaro A, Bracci M, Gesuita R, Carle F, Amati M, Baldassari M, et al. Influence of shift-work on selected immune variables in nurses. Industrial Health. 2011;**49**(5):597-604

[118] Wegrzyn LR, Tamimi RM, Rosner BA, Brown SB, Stevens RG, Eliassen AH, et al. Rotating night-shift work and the risk of breast cancer in the nurses' health studies. American Journal of Epidemiology. 2017;**186**:532-540

[119] Jehan S, Zizi F, Pandi-Perumal SR, Myers AK, Auguste E, Jean-Louis G, et al. Shift work and sleep: Medical implications and management. Sleep Medicine and Disorders. 2017;**1**:00008

[120] Rosa D, Terzoni S, Dellafiore F, Destrebecq A. Systematic review of shift work and nurses' health. Occupational Medicine. 2019;**69**:237-243

[121] Alimoglu MK, Donmez L. Daylight exposure and the other predictors of burnout among nurses in a university hospital. International Journal of Nursing Studies. 2005;**42**:549-555

[122] Caruso CC. Reducing risks to women linked to shift work, long work hours, and related workplace sleep and fatigue issues. Journal of Women's Health. 2015;**24**:789-794

Chapter 10

# Effect of a Video-Supported Nurse-Led Advance Care Planning for Older Adults with Frailty: A Randomized Controlled Trial

*Doris Y.P. Leung, Helen Y.L. Chan, Patrick K.C. Chiu and Raymond S.K. Lo*

### Abstract

This chapter reports the results of a parallel, double-blinded randomized controlled trial to examine the effect of video-supported nurse-led advance care planning (ACP) as compared with a health education program plus an ACP promotion leaflet on end-of-life decision-making outcomes in older adults with frailty. Outcomes were assessed at 1 month and 6 months after the intervention via telephone. Between December 2018 and January 2020, 449 older adults were screened for eligibility. The trial was terminated early after 105 subjects had been assigned (intervention: 51; control: 54) because of the COVID-19 pandemic and the end of the funding period. No significant between-group difference was found in the retention rate at 1 (41.2% vs. 38.9%) and 6 months (35.3% vs. 44.4%). In the intention-to-treat analysis, the ACP group reported a higher but non-significant advance directive completion rate (5.9% vs. 1.9%) and a significantly higher mean score in quality of communication about end-of-life care at 1 month estimated difference: 8.73 (1.16–16.30). There was no evidence of a difference in favorable outcomes of subjects receiving the video-supported, nurse-led ACP compared with those receiving active control. Results might have been confounded by high attrition, poor intervention completion, and reduced sample size due to the early termination of the study.

**Keywords:** advance care planning, advance directives, decision aids, decision-making, end-of-life communication, frailty, older adult

## 1. Introduction

End-of-life (EOL) care has been defined as care "to assist patients who are facing imminent or distant death to have a quality of life possible till the end of their life regardless of their medical diagnosis, health condition or ages" [1]. EOL care encompasses not only the provision of medical support but also social, emotional, and spiritual support [2]. Discussing EOL care can help create a shared understanding of the patient'ss values and care preferences, which can lead to a plan of care that is congruent with these values and preferences [3].

Advance care planning (ACP) is a process of communication aimed at helping individuals proactively make decisions on their EOL care when they are mentally competent [4]. Previous studies consistently reported that ACP is beneficial to patients, family members, healthcare professionals, and the healthcare system. With honest and open ACP conversations, a better understanding of patient's wishes and preferences is gained, thereby increasing their satisfaction with the care that they receive [5, 6]. Other studies found that early ACP conversations lead to the avoidance of aggressive medication interventions, which can improve the patient's quality of life and help family members adjust to their bereavement [7, 8]. ACP can also facilitate healthcare professionals' understanding of patient's goals of care; thus, healthcare professionals can be more certain about what action to offer [9]. Having early ACP can lead to better utilization of healthcare resources. It has resulted in a reduction in hospitalizations and in the increased use of hospice and palliative care services [10, 11]. A recent systematic review of 132 randomized controlled trials (RCTs) concluded that ACP interventions improve patient outcomes including quality of patient-physician communication, preference for comfort care, decisional conflict, patient–caregiver congruence in preference, and ACP documentation [12].

Frailty has been referred to as a complex chronic condition where patients experience more than one chronic illness, have a deceased ability to engage independently in the activities of daily living and are at an increased risk of morbidity and mortality [13, 14]. A recent systematic review of population-level studies from 62 countries across the world estimated that 12% of older adults are suffering from frailty [15]. Thus, ACP is especially important for older patients with frailty. Previous studies summarized EOL care needs of older adults with frailty, which included domains in physical health (e.g., pain management), psychosocial needs, functional status, care-related outcome (e.g., satisfaction with care), and preference of care [16, 17]. Frailty generally causes gradual and slow progression of decline, creating difficulty for healthcare professionals to predict patients' prognosis and identify their EOL phase, especially for frail patients who do not have a recognized life-limiting illness [18]. As a result of the unpredictable prognosis in patients with frailty, there are calls for initiating ACP conversations to discuss goals of care and preferences to make advance care plans in these patients. Having these conversations may increase patient's awareness of the benefits of palliative care [19].

However, technical medical terms, such as cardiopulmonary resuscitation (CPR), antibiotics, and intravenous infusion, are to be covered when discussing common treatment options for EOL care in the ACP conversations. The procedures for these medical treatments are usually described in an abstract, hypothetical way, but the related content may not be understandable for laymen, especially those with limited health literacy. Meta-analytic evidence showed that video-based interventions present a promising way to promote patient's preferences for these EOL care treatment options and knowledge related to ACP but not in the completion of advance directives (AD) [20]. Thus, the addition of a video on EOL care treatment options to support clinical communication in the ACP conversation can further enhance the quality of ACP conversations in EOL care communication.

The aim of the study was to compare the effectiveness of two structured ACP programs with different intensities (one focuses on communication and AD with video decision aids, whilst the other focuses on AD promotion only) on EOL decision outcomes of older adults with frailty and their carers. In this chapter, we only report results from the patients because the sample size for carers was too small for analysis.

## 2. Methods

### 2.1 Study design and participants

The trial was a parallel, double-blinded, prospective RCT with blinded assessment at 1-month and 6-month follow-up conducted at one geriatric medical ward in Hong Kong. The trial protocol was approved by the research ethics committees of the participating hospital and the university of the principal investigator. Written informed consent was obtained from all the participants and family members who joined the study. Participants were assured their right to withdraw from the study at any time without reprisal. The method and protocol of the trial have been reported elsewhere [21].

We recruited eligible subjects at a medical ward of a public hospital in Hong Kong using convenience sampling. The participating hospital is a major hospital providing geriatric medicine and palliative medicine service in the serving district. Hospital nurses referred potentially eligible patients who were about to be discharged to our research assistant (RA1) for eligibility screening. Eligible patients were invited to join the study with signed written consent after an explanation. The inclusion criteria for patients were (1) in-patients, (2) 60 years old or above, (3) fulfilling at least one criterion of the FRAIL scale [22], (4) being clinically stable, (5) able to communicate in Chinese, and (6) cognitively intact (mini-mental state examination [MMSE] > 17) [23]. The exclusion criteria were patients who (1) had already signed an AD or (2) had been referred to a palliative care service during the study period. Consented patients were then asked to nominate an informal caregiver who would likely be a substitute decision-maker for them in future health care. RA1 then approached the nominated caregiver and explained the study to him/her. The inclusion criteria for caregivers were (1) 18 years old or above and (2) able to communicate in Chinese. We recruited patient-caregiver dyads in which patients could join without a caregiver but caregivers could not join without a corresponding patient in the study.

### 2.2 Randomization and masking

Randomization was conducted based on a 1:1 ratio for each treatment arm. A statistician who was not involved in subject recruitment and data collection generated the random allocation list using a computer-generated randomizer. Allocation concealment was implemented by the use of sealed envelopes. Each consented dyad was randomly assigned to either the intervention group to receive a video-supported, nurse-led ACP program or the control group to receive a health education program plus a leaflet promoting ACP after completing the baseline assessment. The envelope was opened by RA1. After randomization, RA1 scheduled the first home visit within 1 week with the participants and sent the participants' information to the nurse who was responsible for the delivery of the corresponding treatment accordingly, with RN1 delivering the ACP intervention and RN2 responsible for the health education program. This procedure can ensure that both the interventionists (RN1 and RN2) were blinded to group allocation. Given that both treatment groups cover ACP elements to a different extent, the participants should also be blinded to their group allocation.

### 2.3 Intervention material

The interventions for the two groups followed the published study protocol [21]. The two structured ACP interventions had two 1-h sessions and were delivered at the patient's home on a weekly basis.

For the intervention group (ACP), participants (the patient and caregivers, if any) received a video-supported, nurse-led ACP program developed using the patient-centered approach. The home-based ACP program involved two 1-h sessions covering four main elements: understanding illness; values and beliefs about care preferences; health prognosis of the disease; and introducing the idea and arrangement of AD. In addition, a 3-min video covering treatment options of EOL care in Hong Kong was shown when discussing health prognosis of disease in the ACP conversations. A personal workbook on ACP was provided to summarize the ACP conversations for participants' records. The nurse who delivered the program had more than 5 years of clinical experience and was trained to facilitate the ACP conversation in a 2-day training workshop.

For the control group (control), participants received a health education program about specific symptoms or diseases provided by another nurse. A leaflet about ADs with contact information for signing AD was distributed at the end of the second session.

### 2.4 Data collection

After obtaining written consent, baseline data were collected by RA1. RA1 then randomly assigned the consented participants to either the control or the intervention group by opening the sealed envelope. Participants were followed up at 1 and 6 months after intervention via telephone by another trained RA2 who was blinded to group allocation. A designated private physician was recruited for AD completion in the study.

### 2.5 Outcome measures

Details of primary and secondary outcomes were described in the published study protocol [21]. In brief, completion of AD was the primary outcome. Those patients who were willing to sign an AD was referred to a designated private physician for completion. The AD form used in the study was adapted from a previous version of the modified directive model by the Hong Kong Hospital Authority [21, 24] with permission.

We also collected data on the following three secondary outcomes from patients and reported their results in the chapter. (1) Patients' decisional conflict in making decisions related to future care was measured by the SURE test [25]. The SURE test has four items in a "Yes/No" format, and its total score can range from 0 to 4, with higher scores indicating higher levels of certainty regarding decision-making. (2) The quality of communication on EOL care with healthcare professionals was measured with the subscale "quality of communication about end-of-life care" (QoC-EOL) of the quality of communication questionnaire developed by Engelberg and colleagues [26, 27]. The subscale has seven items measuring a participant's perception of quality of the ACP communication on an 11-point Likert scale ranging from 0 (the very worst I could imagine) to 10 (the very best I could imagine). There are two additional options for selection: "didn't have the related communication" and "don't know" (to indicate that they were unsure of how to rate the facilitator on a particular skill). For QoC-EOL, we imputed "0" for the two additional options based on the assumption that the failure to complete or address an item warranted a low score because all of the included items were identified as important aspects of EOL care communication [27]. Scores of the seven in the scale were summed up to create the total score with a possible range of 0–70. (3) Patient's knowledge of ACP (ACP knowledge) was measured by a self-developed knowledge questionnaire consisting of five items covering the purposes of AD, EOL discussion, and issues related to ACP. The ACP knowledge score can range from 0 to 5, with higher scores indicating better knowledge. Good content validity (CVI > 0.9) and internal consistency (0.84) were obtained based on the data from a previous local study [28]. At the 1-month follow-up, patient's satisfaction with the treatment received was measured by an item on a 0–10 VAS scale. In addition, intervention patients were asked to rate their comfort level of watching the 3-min video on treatment options of EOL care on a 0–10 VAS scale.

### 2.6 Statistical analysis

The analysis was conducted on the intention-to-treat population whenever applicable. The sample size calculation was based on the primary outcome of AD completion, with a power of 80% at a 5% level of significance using a chi-square test and a 20% attrition rate at 6 months to detect a difference of 14.8% (16.5% for the intervention group and 1.7% for the control group) [28]. After the start of subject recruitment, the required sample size was revised from 298 to 148, with approval from the funding body because of computational error in the original calculation.

Demographic data were summarized and compared with the group difference at baseline by using chi-square tests for categorical variables and Mann–Whitney U tests for continuous variables. For the primary outcome variable, we compared the proportion of AD completion between the intervention and the control group using Fisher's exact test. We used the Mann–Whitney U test to compare the SURE, QoC-EOL, and ACP knowledge score changes between groups, as well as to compare their scores at 1 and 6 months between groups. Furthermore, we conducted generalized estimating equations (GEEs) to examine the differences in the mean changes between the two groups in the secondary outcomes, with adjustment for imbalances in characteristics at baseline. The interaction term of group by time was included to assess the corresponding changes in the outcome variable at the follow-up time points with respect to baseline. All statistical tests, performed using SPSS version 26.0 (IBM Corp., Armonk, NY, USA), were two-sided, and $p < 0.05$ was considered statistically significant. This trial was registered with Chinese Clinical Trial Registry ChiCTR-IOR-17012341.

## 3. Results

### 3.1 Subject recruitment and characteristics

Between December 2018 and January 2020, we assessed 449 patients for trial eligibility. However, subject recruitment was suspended since January 2020 due to the outbreak of the COVID-19 pandemic, leading to the cessation of all research activities in the study hospital and home-based intervention delivery in the RCT. The RCT was terminated prematurely by May 2022 due to the end of funding after two extensions of the study period. During this period, a total of 143 (31.8%) older adults with frailty were eligible for study inclusion, and 105 (73.4%) provided informed consent and were enrolled in the RCT, with 51 allocated to the ACP group and 54 to the control group (**Figure 1**). Of the 51 patients in the ACP group, 40 (78.4%) patients joined the study without caregivers and 11 had caregivers. During the study period, 33 had received the ACP intervention, 20 refused to receive the intervention (mostly because of the social event in 2019 in Hong Kong), 1 passed away and 5 were pending for intervention due to the COVID-19 situation. Video on treatment options of EOL care was shown in 30 cases in the ACP group (90.9%). No adverse event was reported during the sensitive discussion in the ACP conversations. Of the 54 patients in the control group, 39 (72.2%) of them joined the study without caregivers and 15 had caregivers, and 31 (57.4%) had received the health education program, 8 refused, 10

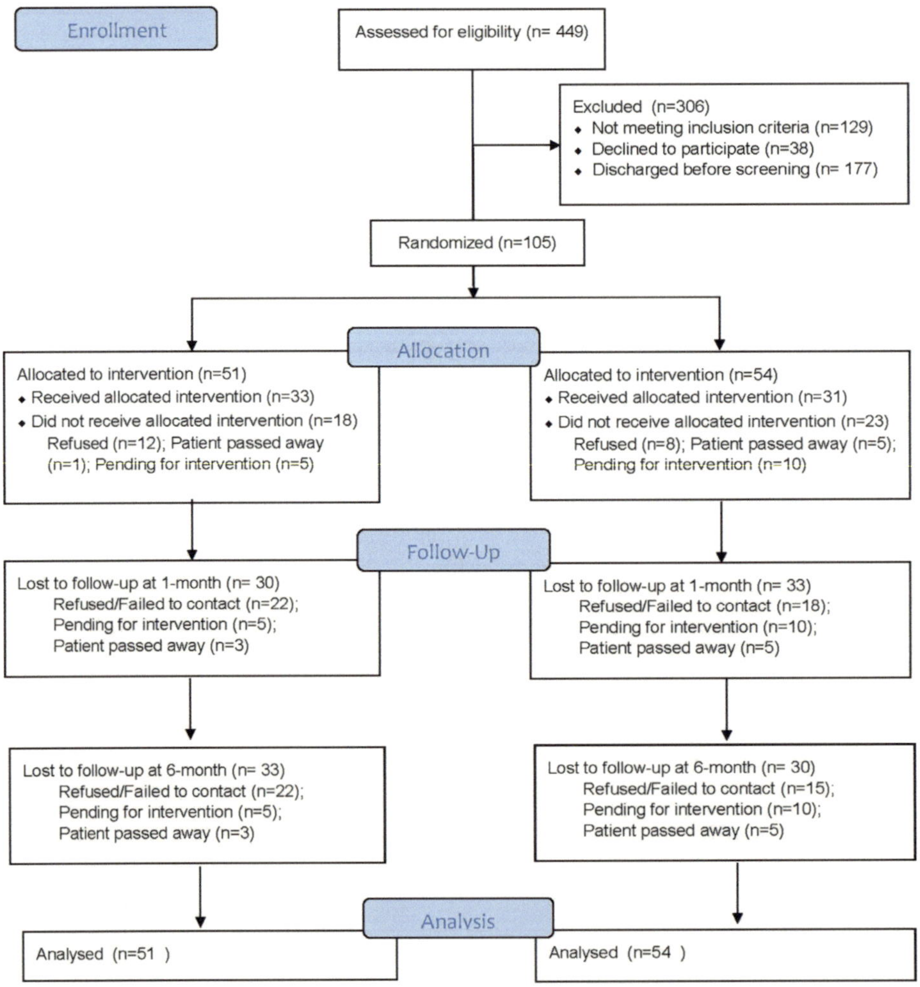


**Figure 1.**
*Flow diagram of the trial.*

were pending intervention, and 5 passed away. The overall attrition rate was 60.0% at both follow-up time points, and there was no statistical difference in the attrition rate between the two groups at 1 (ACP: 58.8% vs. Control: 61.1%, p = 0.819) and 6 months (64.7% vs. 55.6%, p = 0.344).

Baseline patient characteristics are presented in **Table 1**. The study sample included mainly males (62.9%, n = 66), married (60.0%, n = 63), not living alone (81.9%, n = 86), had religion (56.2%, n = 59), and had primary education or below (52.4%, n = 55). The patients had a median (interquartile range [IQR]) age of 82.0 (74.0, 85.0) years and a median MMSE score of 24.0 (21.0, 27.0). On the basis of the possible range of 8–24, the patients reported high levels of daily activities of living with a median of 20.0 (16.0, 23.0) and instrumental daily activities of living with a median of 16.0 (10.5, 22.0). Baseline characteristics were generally balanced in the study sample, except for the FRAIL score, in which the ACP group patients were less frail with a median of 2.0 (1.0, 3.0) than the control group patients whose median was 3.0 (2.0, 4.0), with a p-value of 0.006. For the secondary outcome variables, all the patients in the sample reported extremely low scores in all three secondary outcomes at baseline: QoC-EOL with a median of 0 (0.0, 0.0), SURE with a median of 0.0 (0.0, 3.0) and ACP knowledge with a median of 1.0 (1.0, 2.0).

**Table 2** shows the bivariate analysis results, and **Table 3** illustrates the logistic regression results for the primary outcomes and GEE results for the secondary outcomes of the trial, with the adjustment for FRAIL score at baseline and whether the patients had received the assigned group treatment. For the primary outcome, we found no evidence of a difference in the proportion of patients who had signed an AD during the study period (3 [5.9%] of 51 patients in the ACP group vs. 1 [1.9%] of 54 in the control group, odds ratio [OR] 3.31, 95% CI (0.33, 32.93). The result remained unchanged after adjusting for the effects of baseline FRAIL score and whether the patients had completed the allocated treatment (adjusted OR 3.32, 95% CI (0.33, 32.79); **Tables 2** and **3**).

For the perceived quality of communication on EOL care, the median (IQR) in QoC-EOL score at 1 month was 15.0 (0.0, 22.0) in the ACP group and 0.0 (0.0, 12.0) in the control group. The difference in the median score at 1 month between the two groups was statistically significant (p = 0.048), but the significant result diminished at 6 months. The median (IQR) score in QoC-EOL at 6 months was 0.0 (0.0, 7.0) in the ACP group and 0.0 (0.0, 0.0) in the control group. The median (IQR) change in the QoC-EOL score from baseline to 1 month was 10.0 (0.0, 22.0) in the ACP group and 0.0 (0.0, 12.0) in the control group, whilst the median change from baseline to 6 months was 0.0 (0.0, 6.3) in the ACP group and 0.0 (0.0, 0.0) in the control group. Mann–Whitney U test results showed no evidence of differences in the median change in QoC-EOL at both follow-up time points (**Table 2**). However, we observed a significant between-group difference in the change in QoC-EOL score. Patients in the ACP group reported a higher QoC-EOL score at 1 month than those in the control group, with an estimated mean difference (95% CI) of 8.73 (1.16, 16.30) after controlling for the effects of baseline FRAIL score and whether the patients had received the allocated treatment in GEE analysis (**Table 3**).

For decisional conflict, the two groups exhibited an increase in SURE score to a similar extent, with a median of 1.0 at 1 month and 4.0 at 6 months (p-values >0.8). The median (IQR) change from baseline to 1 month was 0.5 (−0.8, 1.8) in the ACP group and 0.0 (−1.0, 0.0) in the control group, and that from baseline to 6 months was 3.0 (0.0, 3.0) in the ACP group and 1.0 (−0.5, 2.5) in the control group (**Table 2**). The GEE results also supported that there was no evidence of differences in the mean

| | Total (n = 105) | ACP (n = 51) | Control (n = 54) | p-value |
|---|---|---|---|---|
| **Demographic characteristics** | | | | |
| Gender | | | | 0.982 |
| Male | 66 (62.9) | 32 (62.7) | 34 (63.0) | |
| Female | 39 (37.1) | 19 (37.3) | 20 (37.0) | |
| Education | | | | 0.980 |
| Some education | 24 (22.9) | 12 (23.5) | 12 (22.2) | |
| Primary | 31 (29.5) | 16 (31.4) | 15 (27.8) | |
| Secondary | 32 (30.5) | 15 (29.4) | 17 (31.5) | |
| Tertiary or above | 15 (14.3) | 7 (13.7) | 8 (14.8) | |
| Missing data | 3 (2.9) | 1 (2.0) | 2 (3.7) | |
| Marital status | | | | 0.828 |
| Married | 63 (60.0) | 29 (56.9) | 34 (63.0) | |
| Single | 9 (8.6) | 4 (7.8) | 5 (9.3) | |
| Widowed | 30 (28.6) | 16 (31.4) | 14 (25.9) | |
| Divorced | 3 (2.9) | 2 (3.9) | 1 (1.9) | |
| Living alone | | | | 0.696 |
| Yes | 19 (18.1) | 10 (19.6) | 9 (16.7) | |
| No | 86 (81.9) | 41 (80.4) | 45 (83.3) | |
| Had religion | | | | 0.893 |
| Yes | 59 (56.2) | 29 (56.9) | 30 (55.6) | |
| No | 46 (43.8) | 22 (43.1) | 24 (44.4) | |
| Age (years) | 82.0 (74.0, 85.0) | 81.0 (75.0, 84.0) | 82.0 (73.0, 86.3) | 0.546 |
| MMSE score | 24.0 (21.0, 27.0) | 25.0 (21.0, 26.0) | 24.0 (21.0, 27.0) | 0.611 |
| FRAIL score | 3.0 (2.0, 3.0) | 2.0 (1.0, 3.0) | 3.0 (2.0, 4.0) | *0.006* |
| ADL score | 20.0 (16.0, 23.0) | 22.0 (16.0, 24.0) | 20.0 (15.8, 23.0) | 0.395 |
| IADL score | 16.0 (10.5, 22.0) | 16.0 (10.0, 23.0) | 16.0 (10.8, 21.0) | 0.604 |
| **Secondary outcome** | | | | |
| QoC-EOL score | 0.0 (0.0, 0.0) | 0.0 (0.0, 0.0) | 0.0 (0.0, 0.0) | 0.865 |
| SURE score | 0.0 (0.0, 3.0)[a] | 0.0 (0.0, 3.0) | 0.0 (0.0, 3.0)[a] | 0.949 |
| ACP Knowledge score | 1.0 (1.0, 2.0)[c] | 2.0 (1.0, 2.5)[b] | 1.0 (1.0, 2.0)[b] | 0.429 |

*Note: Data are n (%) or median (Interquartile range). MMSE = Mini-Mental State Examination; QoC-EOL: Quality of communication about end-of-life care; [a] Data of 1 patient was missing; [b] Data of 2 patients were missing; [c] Data of 4 patients were missing.*

**Table 1.**
*Patient demographic characteristics and secondary outcome measures at baseline.*

change in the SURE scores from baseline to 1 month and to 6 months in the two groups after controlling for the effect of baseline FRAIL score and whether they had received the allocated treatment (**Table 3**).

For ACP knowledge, the control group exhibited higher median scores than the ACP group at both 1 and 6 months. However, the median change in ACP knowledge was 0 in both groups from baseline to 1 month, whereas the median (IQR) change

| Outcome | ACP | Control | p-value |
|---|---|---|---|
| **Primary outcome** | | | |
| AD completion | 3 (5.9%; n = 51) | 1 (1.9%; n = 54) | 0.281 |
| **Secondary outcome** | | | |
| QoC-EoL score | | | |
| at 1 month | 15.0 (0.0, 22.0; n = 21) | 0.0 (0.0, 12.0; n = 21) | *0.048* |
| at 6 months | 0.0 (0.0, 7.0; n = 18) | 0.0 (0.0, 0.0; n = 24) | 0.271 |
| from baseline to 1 month | 10.0 (0.0, 22.0; n = 21) | 0.0 (0.0, 12.0; n = 21) | 0.194 |
| from baseline to 6 months | 0.0 (0.0, 6.3; n = 18) | 0.0 (0.0, 0.0; n = 24) | 0.599 |
| SURE score | | | |
| at 1 month | 1.0 (0.0, 2.8; n = 20) | 1.0 (0.0, 2.0; n = 19) | 0.828 |
| at 6 months | 4.0 (2.0, 4.0; n = 9) | 4.0 (2.0, 4.0; n = 6) | 0.888 |
| from baseline to 1 month | 0.5 (−0.8, 1.8; n = 20) | 0.0 (−1.0, 0.0; n = 19) | 0.338 |
| from baseline to 6 months | 3.0 (0.0, 3.0; n = 9) | 1.0 (−0.5, 2.5; n = 6) | 0.504 |
| ACP knowledge | | | |
| at 1 month | 1.0 (1.0, 3.0; n = 21) | 1.5 (1.0, 2.0; n = 20) | 0.955 |
| at 6 months | 1.0 (0.8, 3.3; n = 14) | 2.0 (1.0, 3.0; n = 12) | 0.693 |
| from baseline to 1 month | 0.0 (−1.0, 1.0; n = 21) | 0.0 (0.0, 1.8; n = 20) | 0.262 |
| from baseline to 6 months | 0.0 (−1.0, 1.0; n = 13) | 0.5 (−0.8, 2.0; n = 12) | 0.130 |

*Note: Data are n (%) or median (Interquartile range). QoC-EOL: Quality of communication about end-of-life care.*

**Table 2.**
*Primary and secondary outcomes.*

| Outcome | Adjusted OR (95%CI) | p-value |
|---|---|---|
| **AD completion** | 3.32 (0.33–32.79) | 0.307 |
| | Beta coefficient (95%CI) | p-value |
| **QoC-EOL** | | |
| Group | | |
| ACP | 0.29 (−0.66, 1.24) | 0.549 |
| Control | Reference | |
| Time | | |
| Baseline | Reference | |
| 1 month | 5.89 (1.79, 9.99) | *0.005* |
| 6 months | 1.28 (−0.98, 3.54) | 0.267 |
| Group x Time interaction | | |
| ACP x 1 month | 8.73 (1.16, 16.30) | *0.024* |
| ACP x 6 months | 1.29 (−5.70, 8.28) | 0.717 |
| **SURE** | | |
| Group | | |
| ACP | −0.03 (−0.65, 0.60) | 0.930 |

| Outcome | Adjusted OR (95%CI) | p-value |
|---|---|---|
| Control | Reference | |
| Time | | |
| Baseline | Reference | |
| 1 month | 0.09 (−0.51, 0.69) | 0.769 |
| 6 months | 0.78 (−0.65, 2.21) | 0.286 |
| Group x Time interaction | | |
| ACP x 1 month | 0.22 (−0.76, 1.21) | 0.657 |
| ACP x 6 months | 0.42 (−1.25, 2.08) | 0.623 |
| **ACP Knowledge** | | |
| Group | | |
| ACP | 0.14 (−0.30, 0.57) | 0.538 |
| Control | Reference | |
| Time | | |
| Baseline | Reference | |
| 1 month | 0.32 (−0.23, 0.87) | 0.257 |
| 6 months | 0.53 (−0.23, 1.28) | 0.175 |
| Group x Time interaction | | |
| ACP x 1 month | −0.15 (−0.98, 0.68) | 0.727 |
| ACP x 6 months | −0.70 (−1.76, 0.35) | 0.191 |

*Note: CI = confidence interval; FRAIL score and completion of intervention were added in the models.*

**Table 3.**
*Results of logistic regression on primary outcome and generalized estimating equations on secondary outcomes.*

from baseline to 6 months remained at 0 (−1.0, 1.0) in the ACP group and was increased by 0.5 (−0.8, 2.0) in the control group (**Table 2**). The GEE results showed that the mean values of ACP knowledge remained stable in the two groups over time, and there was no evidence of a difference in the mean changes in the ACP knowledge score between the two groups at both 1-month and 6-month follow-up (**Table 3**).

Amongst the 64 patients who completed 1-month follow-up, the level of satisfaction with the received treatment was high in both the intervention group (median [IQR]) (8.0 [5.3, 10.0], n = 33) and the control group (8.0 [5.0, 10.0], n = 31), with no statistically significant difference between the groups ($p = 1.0$). For the 30 interventional patients who had watched the 3-min video on EOL care treatment options, the median (IQR) in the comfort level was also high at 7.0 (4.0, 8.0).

## 4. Discussion

On the basis of the prespecified intention-to-treat analysis, the trial did not show a benefit of the video-supported nurse-led ACP program over the health education program plus an ACP promotion leaflet for end-of-life decision-making outcomes. However, our results might have been confounded by the poor implementation of the study because of three reasons: (1) the slowing down of research activities due to the social event in 2019 in Hong Kong, (2) the complete halt of all research activities due to the outbreak of the COVID-19 pandemic in January 2020, and (3) end of the funding period of the study, which eventually led to the early termination of the trial. These events limited our final sample size to only 105 (70.9%) of our planned target of 148 patients, together with the large attrition rates in the two follow-up time points in both groups, resulting in an underpowered analysis. Moreover, the fact that one-third of the patients were not screened for eligibility before discharge might have introduced selection biases that contributed to our observed findings.

In this study, the completion rates of AD in both treatment groups were low compared with previous RCTs, with a range of 0–37.9% in the intervention group and 0.4–23.9% in the control group [29]. The recent systematic reviews on the efficacy of ACP based on 132 RCTs concluded that it improved ACP documentation, with 34 out of 54 included studies (63%) showing significant and positive results [12]. However, amongst these 54 RCTs, only three were conducted in Asian countries [28, 30, 31]. Together with a more recent RCT in Singapore, mixed results on ACP/AD documentation were found: two showed significant improvement in the outcome [28, 30], and the other two had non-significant results [31, 32]. Compared with our previous RCT on ACP conducted in Hong Kong with significant results on ACP/AD documentation [28], we did not observe a difference in the AD completion rate between the two groups although we have added the 3-min video decision aid in the ACP intervention in the current study. The mixed results of RCTs could be explained by the difference in the target patient group. The two RCTs with significant results targeting subjects with limited life expectancy (elderly in nursing homes and patients with advanced serious illness and their proxies) and the two with non-significant results included advanced cancer patients and patients visiting primary care clinics. In this study, we included older adults with frailty who were healthy and had long life expectancies; thus, they would be less likely to see the clinical relevance or urgency of ACP conversations [33, 34]. In our qualitative analysis of ACP conversations who did not complete AD after the ACP intervention, we also found that the older adults generally accepted that getting old and becoming frailer is a natural process instead of feeling anxious about death [35]. They believed they were still healthy and reluctant to discuss EOL issues and indicated they would be willing to engage in ACP conversations when they became terminally ill. The RCT in Singapore with primary care patients also indicated that they were too young to consider completion of AD [32]. Discussing death-related issues is still taboo in many Asian cultures [36]. The findings from these RCTs, including the current trial, provide some support regarding the optimal time for ACP in the Asian context: ACP conversations with patients who are not approaching their end of life may be too inappropriate when these patients still consider themselves healthy, although more studies are required to provide a firm conclusion to this assertion. Nevertheless, we clearly need other initiatives that promote EOL discussion in Asian countries. For example, a community action approach to promote early ACP conversation through public education by shifting ACP from a health issue to a "normal" conversion to reduce the negative feeling related to death advocated in the literature could be an option [37].

This work is the first trial in the Asian region examining the effect of an ACP intervention on the quality of communication in EOL care. In our study, we observed a significantly greater increase in the median QoC-EOL score from baseline to 1 month after intervention in the ACP group than those in the control group based on the GEE results. Although subject to a large type 2 error, the observation of the increase in quality of communication was consistent with previous studies reporting that ACP interventions can improve the quality of patient-physician communication [12]. However, in the current study with a range of 0–70, the highest median in the observed QoC-EOL score was 15 at 1 month in the ACP group, which was still extremely low. Despite high acceptable levels of satisfaction with the received treatment in both groups, the low median in QoC-EOL scores in this study reflected that the promotional leaflet alone in the control group and the stand-alone two-session ACP intervention in the intervention group might not be sufficient to improve the quality of the communication. A recent RCT also showed that video-alone intervention does not engage individuals in high-quality ACP [38]. The communication on EOL care was determined to be of low quality in this study because of the rareness of its occurrence. A recent systematic review found a low rate (0–5%) of EOL care communication in hospitalized frail older adults, even though 74–84% of older inpatients with capacity were receptive to ACP [39]. A lack of communication on EOL care between healthcare professionals and older adults with frailty seems to be a worldwide problem. On-going discussions and deliberation with a healthcare provider in promoting patient-physician communication on EOL care are necessary [38].

Similar to QoC-EOL, the increases in SURE scores from baseline to 1 and 6 months were greater in the ACP group than in the control group, but the differences in the changes were not statistically significant. The result was contradictory to the findings from a systematic review of ACP interventions [12] that decisional conflict was reduced significantly in 64% (9) of the 14 RCTs that had assessed this outcome including the previous RCT in Hong Kong [28]. The nonsignificant result might be due to the underpowered feature of the study. Another possible reason is the low level of prognostic awareness in the participants. As reported previously, many of the participating older adults in our study believed they were still healthy, and they would be willing to participate in an EOL conversation when they became terminally ill [35]. Hence, they were not likely to make any decision about their EOL care at the present moment. Previous studies showed that low levels of prognostic awareness are associated with difficulty in initiating conversation in older adults [40]. The three RCTs targeting patients with advanced illnesses in the Asian region that had examined this outcome reported mixed results; two studies that included ACP conversations showed that ACP intervention improved decisional conflict [28, 41], whereas another study that used video/booklet without active counseling showed non-significant results [42]. In addition, a previous study reported that individuals with a high ability to understand health information have low decisional conflict [43]. The low intensity of the ACP conversations in the current study might not be sufficient to gain and understand EOL care information for our participants who were comparatively healthy, and it might lead to uncertainty in making EOL care-related decisions.

Conversely, participants in the ACP group reported no change in their ACP-related knowledge median scores after the intervention, whereas those in the control group reported a slight increase in the median scores at 1 and 6 months after the intervention. There was no statistical difference in the changes in ACP knowledge, but the trend of the changes favored the control group. Although we did not have any particular explanation for such an observation, we suspected that this observation might be because of the measurement tool itself. The ACP knowledge has five items with good content validity and internal consistency; however, other psychometric properties, such as factorial and construct validities, have not yet been tested [21]. Thus, the current findings might be subject to measurement error. We recommend that the psychometric properties of the scale be fully examined before its use.

Our study had limitations. The main study limitation was that the trial did not meet recruitment goals, and the analysis was underpowered. The small sample size was a consequence of unexpected events of the social event in 2019 in Hong Kong and the COVID-19 pandemic since 2020; the former had substantially slowed down, and the latter completely hindered all the research activities in the territory. High attrition rates also contributed to the small sample size for analysis. The two follow-up surveys were unavoidably conducted via telephone due to the social event in Hong Kong and the COVID-19 pandemic during the study period that had made face-to-face administration of the questionnaire impossible, even though we realized that the participating older adults could not hear well on the phone and tended to provide missing data. Future studies should consider the face-to-face mode for data collection with older adults with frailty. Another limitation was the arrangement of the completion of AD with a designated private physician. Given that the participants of the study targeted older adults with frailty, it would be troublesome for them to pay an extra visit to the clinic of the private physician to sign the AD even if they were willing to do so. There are many barriers to such a visit, including transportation, traveling fee, and companion for the trip. Although we were willing to provide support to these three barriers for the visit, it became impossible because of the social event in 2019 and the location of the clinic.

## 5. Conclusions

In conclusion, in our trial, a video-supported, nurse-led ACP intervention did not significantly increase the completion of ADs in older adults with frailty who were discharged from hospital in Hong Kong. The optimal time for ACP conversations with Chinese older adults with frailty depends largely on personal perception of health, which deserves further studies.

## Acknowledgements

The research was funded by a grant from the Research Grants Council of the Hong Kong Special Administrative Region, China (grant number PolyU14162617H). Contact: https://www.ugc.edu.hk/. The funding party played no role in the design of the study, the collection, and interpretation of the data, or in the writing of the manuscript.

## Conflict of interest

The authors declare no conflict of interest.

## Notes/thanks/other declarations

We would like to thank the patients and their family members who participated in the project, especially during the COVID-19 pandemic period.

## Author details

Doris Y.P. Leung[1*], Helen Y.L. Chan[2], Patrick K.C. Chiu[3] and Raymond S.K. Lo[4]

1 The Hong Kong Polytechnic University, Hong Kong, China

2 The Chinese University of Hong Kong, Hong Kong, China

3 The University of Hong Kong, Hong Kong, China

4 Shatin Hospital, Hong Kong, China

*Address all correspondence to: doris.yp.leung@polyu.edu.hk

## References

[1] Izumi S, Nagae H, Sakurai C, Imamura E. Defining end-of-life care from perspectives of nursing ethics. Nursing Ethics. 2012;**19**(5):608-618. DOI: 10.1177/0969733011436205

[2] Driessen A, Borgstrom E, Cohn S. Placing death and dying: Making place at the end of life. Social Science & Medicine. 2021;**291**:113974. DOI: 10.1016/j.socscimed.2021.113974

[3] Sinuff T, Dodek P, You JJ, Barwich D, Tayler C, Downar J, et al. Improving end-of-life communication and decision making: The development of a conceptual framework and quality indicators. Journal of Pain and Symptom Management. 2015;**49**(6):1071-1080. DOI: 10.1016/j.jpainsymman.2014.12.007

[4] Rietjens JAC, Sudore RL, Connolly M, van Delden JJ, Drickamer MA, Droger M, et al. European association for palliative care. Definition and recommendations for advance care planning: An international consensus supported by the European Association for palliative care. Lancet Oncology. 2017;**18**(9):e543-e551. DOI: 10.1016/S1470-2045(17)30582-X

[5] Gonella S, Basso I, Clari M, Di Giulio P. A qualitative study of family carers views on how end-of-life communication contributes to palliative-oriented care in nursing home. Annali dell'Istituto superiore di sanita. 2020;**56**(3):315-324. DOI: 10.4415/ANN_20_03_09

[6] You JJ, Dodek P, Lamontagne F, Downar J, Sinuff T, Jiang X, et al. Accept study team and the Canadian researchers at the end of life network (CARENET): What really matters in end-of-life discussions? Perspectives of patients in hospital with serious illness and their families. Canadian Medical Association Journal. 2014;**186**(18):E679-E687. DOI: 10.1503/cmaj.140673

[7] Mack JW, Cronin A, Keating NL, Taback N, Huskamp HA, Malin JL, et al. Associations between end-of-life discussion characteristics and care received near death: A prospective cohort study. Journal of Clinical Oncology. 2012;**30**(35):4387-4395. DOI: 10.1200/JCO.2012.43.6055

[8] Wright AA, Zhang B, Ray A, Mack JW, Trice E, Balboni T, et al. Associations between end-of-life discussions, patient mental health, medical care near death, and caregiver bereavement adjustment. Journal of the American Medical Association. 2008;**300**(14):1665-1673. DOI: 10.1001/jama.300.14

[9] Fulmer T, Escobedo M, Berman A, Koren MJ, Hernández S, Hult A. Physicians' views on advance care planning and end-of-life care conversations. Journal of the American Geriatric Society. 2018;**66**(6):1201-1205. DOI: 10.1111/jgs.15374

[10] Brinkman-Stoppelenburg A, Rietjens JA, van der Heide A. The effects of advance care planning on end-of-life care: A systematic review. Palliative Medicine. 2014;**28**(8):1000-1025. DOI: 10.1177/0269216314526272

[11] Martin RS, Hayes B, Gregorevic K, Lim WK. The Effects of advance care planning interventions on nursing home residents: A systematic review. Journal of the American Medical Directors Association. 2016;**17**(4):284-293. DOI: 10.1016/j.jamda.2015.12.017

[12] Malhotra C, Shafiq M, Batcagan-Abueg APM. What is the evidence

for efficacy of advance care planning in improving patient outcomes? A systematic review of randomized controlled trial. BMJ Open. 2022;**12**:e060201. DOI: 10.1136/bmjopen-2021-060201

[13] Abbasi M, Rolfson D, Khera AS, Dabravolskaj J, Dent E, Xia L. Identification and management of frailty in the primary care setting. Canada Medical Association Journal. 2018;**190**(38):e1134-e1140. DOI: 10.1503/cmaj.171509 Erratum in: Canada Medical Association Journal. 2019;191(2):e54

[14] Carter C, Leanza F, Mohammed S, Upshur R, Kontos P. A rapid scoping review of end-of-life conversations with frail older adults in Canada. Canadian Family Physician. 2021;**67**(11):e298-e305. DOI: 10.46747/cfp.6711e298

[15] O'Caoimh R, Sezgin D, O'Donovan MR, Molloy DW, Clegg A, Rockwood K, et al. Prevalence of frailty in 62 countries across the world: a systematic review and meta-analysis of population-level studies. Age and Ageing. 2021;**50**(1):96-104. DOI: 10.1093/ageing/afaa219

[16] Crooms RC, Gelfman LP. Palliative care and end-of-life considerations for the frail patient. Anesthesia and Analgesia. 2020;**130**(6):1504-1515. DOI: 10.1213/ANE.0000000000004763

[17] Stow D, Spiers G, Matthews FE, Hanratty B. What is the evidence that people with frailty have needs for palliative care at the end of life? A systematic review and narrative synthesis. Palliative Medicine. 2019;**33**(4):399-414. DOI: 10.1177/0269216319828650

[18] Cohen-Mansfield J, Skornick-Bouchbinder M, Brill S. Trajectories of end of life: A systematic review. The Journals of Gerontology, Series B, Psychological Sciences and Social Sciences. 2018;**73**(4):564-572. DOI: 10.1093/geronb/gbx093

[19] Cardona-Morrell M, Lewis E, Suman S, Haywood C, Williams M, Brousseau AA, et al. Recognising older frail patients near the end of life: What next? European Journal of Internal Medicine. 2017;**45**:84-90. DOI: 10.1016/j.ejim.2017.09.026

[20] Jain A, Corriveau S, Quinn K, Gardhouse A, Vegas DB, You JJ. Video decision aids to assist with advance care planning: A systematic review and meta-analysis. British Medical Journal Open. 2015;**5**:e007491. DOI: 10.1136/bmjopen-2014-007491

[21] Leung DYP, Chan HYL, Yau SZM, Chiu PKC, Tang FWK, Kwan JSK. A video-supported nurse-led advance care planning on end-of-life decision-making among frail older patients: Protocol for a randomized controlled trial. Journal of Advanced Nursing. 2019;**75**:1360-1369. DOI: 10.1111/jan.13959

[22] Morley JE, Malmstrom TK, Miller DK. A simple frailty questionnaire (FRAIL) predicts outcomes in middle aged African Americans. Journal of Nutrition, Health & Aging. 2012;**16**:601-608. DOI: 10.1007/s12603-012-0084-2

[23] Fan TW. Brief cognitive mental status tests for psychometric outpatients — A pilot study. Journal of Hong Kong College Psychiatry. 1992;**2**:69-78

[24] Hong Kong Hospital Authority. Sample of advance directives form [Internet]. 2020. Available from: https://www.ha.org.hk/haho/ho/psrm/ADformEng1.pdf [Accessed: 2022-10-17]

[25] Légaré F, Kearing S, Clay K, Gagnon S, D'Amours D, Rousseau M. Are

you SURE?: Assessing patient decisional conflict with a 4-item screening test. Canada Family Physician. 2010;**56**(8):e308-e314

[26] Curtis JR, Engelberg RA, Nielsen EL, Au DH, Patrick DL. Patient-physician communication about end-of-life care for patients with severe COPD. The European Respiratory Journal. 2004;**24**(2):200-205. DOI: 10.1183/09031936.04.00010104

[27] Engelberg R, Downey L, Curtis JR. Psychometric characteristics of a quality of communication questionnaire assessing communication about end-of-life care. Journal of Palliative Medicine. 2006;**9**(5):1086-1098. DOI: 10.1089/jpm.2006.9.1086

[28] Chan HY, Ng JS, Chan KS, Ko PS, Leung DY, Chan CW, et al. Effects of a nurse-led post-discharge advance care planning programme for community-dwelling patients nearing the end of life and their family members: A randomised controlled trial. International Journal of Nursing Studies. 2018;**87**:26-33. DOI: 10.1016/j.ijnurstu.2018.07.008

[29] Houben CHM, Spruit MA, Groenen MT, Wouters EFM, Janssen DJA. Efficacy of advance care planning: A systematic review and meta-analysis. Journal of the American Medical Directors Association. 2014;**15**:477-480. DOI: 10.1016/j.jamda.2014.01.008

[30] Chiu Wu CH, Perng SJ, Shi CK, Lai HL. Advance care planning and advance directives: A multimedia education program in community-dwelling older adults. Journal of Applied Gerontology. 2020;**39**(8):811-819. DOI: 10.1177/0733464819831596

[31] Wen FH, Chen CH, Chou WC, Chen JS, Chang WC, Hsieh CH, et al. Evaluating if an advance care planning intervention promotes do-not-resuscitate orders by facilitating accurate prognostic awareness. Journal of the National Comprehensive Cancer Network. 2020;**18**(12):1658-1666. DOI: 10.6004/jnccn.2020.7601

[32] Xu C, Yan S, Chee J, Lee EPY, Lim HW, Lim SWC, et al. Increasing the completion rate of the advance directives in primary care setting – A randomized controlled trial. BMC Family Practice. 2021;**22**:115. DOI: 10.1186/s12875-021-01473-1

[33] Bernard C, Tan A, Slaven M, Elston D, Heyland DK, Howard M. Exploring patient-reported barriers to advance care planning in family practice. BMC Family Practice. 2020;**21**(1):94. DOI: 10.1186/s12875-020-01167-0

[34] Combes S, Gillett K, Norton C, Nicholson CJ. The importance of living well now and relationships: A qualitative study of the barriers and enablers to engaging frail elders with advance care planning. Palliative Medicine. 2021;**35**(6):1137-1147. DOI: 10.1177/02692163211013260

[35] Wan Z, Chan HYL, Chiu PKC, Lo RSK, Cheng HL, Leung DYP. Experiences of older adults with frailty not completing an advance directive: A qualitative study of ACP conversations. International Journal of Environmental Research and Public Health. 2022;**19**(9):5358. DOI: 10.3390/ijerph19095358

[36] Cheng SY, Lin CP, Chan HY, Martina D, Mori M, Kim SH, et al. Advance care planning in Asian culture. Japanese Journal of Clinical Oncology. 2020;**50**:976-989

[37] McIlfatrick S, Slater P, Bamidele O, Muldrew D, Beck E, Hasson F. It's almost superstition: If I don't think about it,

it won't happen'. Public knowledge and attitudes towards advance care planning: A sequential mixed methods study. Palliative Medicine. 2021;**35**(7):1356-1365. DOI: 10.1177/02692163211015838

[38] Douglas ML, Simon J, Davison SN, Biondo P, Ghosh S, Kassam A, et al. Efficacy of advance care planning videos for patients: A randomized controlled trial in cancer, heart, and kidney failure outpatient settings. Medical Decision Making. 2021;**41**(3):292-304. DOI: 10.1177/0272989X20985836

[39] Hopkins SA, Bentley A, Phillips V, Barclay S. Advance care plans and hospitalized frail older adults: A systematic review. BMJ Supportive & Palliative Care. 2020;**10**(2):164-174. DOI: 10.1136/bmjspcare-2019-002093

[40] Carlini J, Bahudin D, Michaleff ZA, Plunkett E, Shé ÉN, Clark J, et al. Discordance and concordance on perception of quality care at end of life between older patients, caregivers and clinicians: a scoping review. European Geriatric Medicine. 2022;**13**(1):87-99. DOI: 10.1007/s41999-021-00549-6

[41] Malhotra C, Sim D, Jaufeerally FR, Hu M, Nadkarni N, Ng CSH, et al. Impact of a formal advance care planning program on end-of-life care for patients with heart failure: Results from a randomized controlled trial. Journal of Cardiac Failure. 2020;**26**(7):594-598. DOI: 10.1016/j.cardfail.2020.01.015

[42] Yun YH, Kang E, Park S, Koh SJ, Oh HS, Keam B, et al. Efficacy of a decision aid consisting of a video and booklet on advance care planning for advanced cancer patients: Randomized controlled trial. Journal of Pain and Symptom Management. 2019;**58**(6):940-948.e2. DOI: 10.1016/j.jpainsymman.2019.07.032

[43] Pecanac KE, Brown RL, Kremsreiter HB. Decisional conflict during major medical treatment decision-making: A survey study. Journal of General Internal Medicine. 2021;**36**(1):55-61. DOI: 10.1007/s11606-020-06125-1

**Chapter 11**

# Reconceptualizing Geriatric Care in a Sub-Saharan African Context

*Priscilla Yeye Adumoah Attafuah, Cecilia Eliason and Ninon P. Amertil*

## Abstract

Population ageing is very fast catching up worldwide and with a resultant rise in demands for health services and medical costs. This is because older adults are typically more vulnerable to falls and chronic diseases. It is estimated that by 2025, 57% of the world's population aged 80 years or older will be living in less developed regions. By 2050, there is an estimated increase of more than 70%. Although, Africa, on average, has the lowest life expectancy in the world, in virtually every country, the section of people aged 60 years and over is developing faster than any other age group, because of both longer life expectancy and declining fertility rates. Older adults have recommended that nurses should receive some training for improving their behaviour and attitude. Older adults and their significant health needs are different from that of an adult or a child and should be considered to meet SDG Goal 8: "ensuring equitable access to, and utilisation of, health and long-term care services …". Their intense use of health services puts older adults at greater risk of receiving fragmented or poor-quality care. The sheer number of people entering older ages is bound to challenge national structures, particularly health systems. This chapter seeks to review the literature on geriatric health care by specialists.

**Keywords:** geriatric care, geriatric nurses, sub-Saharan Africa, quality of care, gerontology

## 1. Introduction

The former Secretary-General of the United Nations (UN), Kofi Annan, at the second UN World Assembly on Ageing quoted: 'In Africa, it is said that when an old man dies, a library vanishes'. This is because older people in Africa have traditionally been celebrated and respected, although they accounted for a minority of the population. With increasing life expectancy globally and specifically in developing countries, the older adult population constitute a bigger proportion of society than previously. Ashirifi et al. [1] estimate that approximately two-thirds of the world's population aged over 60 years are living in developing countries, and by 2050, 212 million of those will live in Africa. As the ageing population continues to grow exponentially, their demand for hospital care also increases.

## 2. Life expectancy

Across the globe, various initiatives have been put in place to improve the health outcomes of the elderly, to lengthen their life span and decrease the rate of morbidity and mortality of the older adult which in turn increases their numbers among the population [2–4]. The use of comprehensive geriatric assessment (CGA) for assessment, goal setting and care delivery has been adopted in the United Kingdom to improve relational working [5–6]. CGA has been shown to improve outcomes for older people including improved physical and cognitive function, reduced mortality, and readmissions of the elderly to hospitals [6]. Over the years, geriatric care has received a lot of attention, from specialised training of healthcare professionals in the field of practice, to care given to the aged by their families till the end of life [7, 8].

Other factors that have accounted for the increase in the population of older adults in developed countries also include favourable social policies, geriatric care facilities, elderly retirement incentives and insurance schemes to facilitate a comfortable life for the elderly before their demise occurs. All communities in the world are advocating for healthy ageing. The United Nations (UN) and the World Health Organisation (WHO) for several years have been encouraging governments to promote policies aimed at the healthy and successful ageing of their people [9]. Additionally, the American Geriatrics Society (AGS) recently, made recommendations to guide federal, state and local governments in making decisions about the best care for older adults residing in assisted living facilities (ALFs) during the coronavirus disease 2019 (COVID-19) pandemic [10].

## 3. Geriatric care

Geriatric populations are prone to a wide variety of disorders; physical, psychological and social, which require specialised care [11, 12]. Over the years, the maintenance of a healthy body system for the aged has been of utmost importance, with information being sent forth to the public, families and health workers on how to combat physiological, biological, social as well pathological changes among the older adult.

These are all factors that account for the rise in the number of the ageing population across the globe, as their standard of living is improved, prolonging their length of stay as active or thriving members of the world's population. Taking into view some common problems that affect the elderly, several reforms have been made in the health system to fend for the needs of the aged, for example, the guidelines put in place by the National Health Service of the United Kingdom towards the care and surgery of aged patients with hip fractures [13]. A multidisciplinary approach to caring for older adults is highly recommended and in the United Kingdom, national guidelines have been published in this regard. For example, between orthopaedic surgeons and geriatricians in the United Kingdom. This approach to modern hip fracture management aims at achieving the goals of coordinated multidisciplinary care, early surgery and facilitated discharge [13]. Over the years literary works educating the public, families and individuals are published centred on the care of older adults to build upon the public's knowledge of geriatrics.

### 3.1 Age-friendly world

According to the WHO [14], an age-friendly world enables people of all ages to enthusiastically participate in communal activities being treated with respect, irrespective of one's age. An age-friendly world enables older people to be with people they love promoting healthy living and appropriate support for those who can no longer engage in activities of daily living.

In recent years, international organisations and governments have developed age-friendly community models that incorporate aspects of the natural built, and social environment and optimise opportunities for well-being in old age.

Given the growing aged population, the WHO [15] called for special attention to the older adult friendliness of hospitals. Physical aspects of an elder-friendly hospital are defined as features of environmental design including the safety, physical, social and psychological needs of older adults [16–18].

Creating awareness about the need to improve care and support for older people and building agreements within all segments of society on the nature of care and its delivery in the most economical way [19] is vital. In most sub-Saharan countries, older persons are cared for in general wards with no geriatric specialist. However, evidence from developed countries shows this is not healthy for the vulnerable aged population as they have specific needs.

### 3.2 Specialist geriatric care

Internationally, interprofessional education (IPE) models have been used for geriatric syndromes, but not specifically for geriatric health policy. An IPE model has been used in presenting geriatric syndromes, palliative care, dementia care management, teaching the M Framework and fall-risk assessments [20]. IPE offers health profession learners opportunities to learn from, with and about each other. The World Health Organisation recognised IPE in the Ageing 2020 Report proposing that the interprofessional model will ensure optimal health care for the elderly [21].

Amidst the efforts put forth to improve the quality of life of the elderly in society, there are persisting gaps in the number of specialised healthcare professionals in the field. Nurses are recognised as the single largest health service professional who takes care of the aged population [22, 23]. Caring for older people is complex and challenging due to their physical, psychological and social needs. According to the John A. Hartford Foundation [24], there is a scarcity of specialist nurses who take care of older persons, for instance, less than 1% of the 2.56 million registered nurses in the United States, are certified gerontological nurses, and only 3% of the 111,000 advanced practice nurses, are gerontological nurses. In sub-Saharan Africa, this is non-existent. A few geriatric doctors are being trained by the College of Physicians in Ghana but none for the nurses. There is not enough training rendered in primary training institutions. The preparation of future nurses to meet this need is a critical concern for the nursing profession. Currently, there is no dedicated career pathway or exposure to geriatric care in undergraduate nursing programmes in Ghana. Many nurses and doctors have had little if any, specialist education in the care of older people and therefore do not understand the extent of their needs [18].

In some countries, there is still a struggle to provide adequate health facilities needed to meet the health concerns of older adults. Outlined principles for age-friendly hospitals by the WHO [15], include the following (i) Information flow through education, communication and training [training of staff in clinical geriatrics and patient education]; (ii) Healthcare management systems and (iii) Physical environments with clean and comfortable centres that are user friendly irrespective of an individual's age or disability. The number of older patients admitted to acute hospitals has increased; however, with their varying needs, there is no gold-standard method of triaging them towards practising comprehensive geriatric assessment [25]. A recent systematic review of negative health outcomes in older people attending EDs (Emergency Departments) identified adverse events, including under triage of illness severity, lack of recognition of geriatric syndromes, suboptimal drug therapy and adverse communication-related events [26]. Concerns about overcrowding in emergency departments are furthered by the growing population of older adults with increasingly complex healthcare needs. Emergency department (ED) backlogs, and long waits for in-patient beds, diagnostic tests and procedures among older adults. This has raised concerns about patient safety, the timeliness of ED services and the quality of care provided in this acute care treatment setting [27, 28].

Policymakers face a key challenge: how best to allocate fitted resources, improve the quality and fitness for purpose of the workforce, increase recruitment and retention, and ensure efficient ways of working with wider health and social care systems [29].

The publication of a major critique of the neglect of older people in the United States stimulated public concern that led to the creation of the National Institute on Ageing with a multi-million-dollar research budget [30]. Gerontology and geriatrics training in Ghana are limited, but the issues facing the ageing society are enormous due to the limited information available to families. Designing an advanced gerontological system as found in the United States to meet the growing needs of Ghana would be difficult due to the lack of trained professionals and resources [31, 32].

Many strategies can be put up by local governments and health-centred institutions to deal with the persisting gaps. The idea of trying to put up nursing homes and aged facilities is a good idea however a simplified social support system, which is community-based, would be an ideal prototype for providing services to older adults [33]. There is considerable diversity among different communities' needs for specific strategies to become age-friendly. Each approach needs to be rooted in the expressed needs of its residents, both older and younger [34]. One important factor that allows people to age in place comfortably is having the right housing in terms of available facilities, location, size, affordability and tenure [35–37].

## 4. Strategies for a reconceptualisation

In dealing with the gap of the reduced number of health professionals who are specialised in the healthcare of the elderly, supportive initiatives can be put up by the government to build the interest of health workers in the field of gerontology. With the increasing number of older adults in sub-Saharan Africa, it is prudent that nurses require sound gerontological knowledge and skills that permit them to provide quality care to this population. Studies have shown that nurses who are adequately prepared in gerontological nursing, provide quality care which leads to better outcomes [22, 38, 39]. International research evidence suggests a positive association between registered nurse staffing levels and better-quality care and quality of life for nursing home residents [29]. To meet the challenges of building an age-friendly community, policymakers and planners are encouraged to take a proactive approach and engage with multiple stakeholders as well as empower older people themselves to create the conditions for active ageing [40].

The current models of care for frail older adults in sub-Saharan Africa have been heavily hospital-based. Given that hospitals can do more good than harm for frail older adults, this is not unproblematic nonetheless, being cared for by specialist

*DOI: http://dx.doi.org/10.5772/intechopen.109920*

geriatric nurses, will be more appropriate. Additionally, if efforts are made to keep them out of the hospital in the first place (public health nurses trained in geriatric care will play a critical role here), making care less unsafe in the hospital. Furthermore, given current pressures on the NHIS, we must strive to practice health promotion and prevention of diseases rather than curative care. Bringing care closer to people's homes, focusing as much on wellness as on responding to illness [41].

The best way to ensure quality geriatric care is to use evidence-based guidelines and professional standards to guide the practice environment [42]. Nurses consider institutional practices that support the use of evidence-based policies and guidelines, adequate and appropriate resources, administrative commitment and support of specialised geriatric nursing knowledge and skills as essential to quality geriatric care [43]. It is necessary to reconceptualise geriatric care in the African sub-region as this will improve health outcomes among the older adult population leading to an increased life expectancy.

## 5. Conclusions

With the aim of improving the quality of care given to older persons, there is an urgent need to reconceptualise the current geriatric care rendered in sub-Saharan Africa. In view of the numerous evidence from developed countries, of improved outcomes when geriatric health professionals are involved, the African continent can align with the strategies described in this chapter.

## Acknowledgements

We are grateful to the authors of the literature reviewed during the writing of this chapter.

## Conflict of interest

The authors declare no conflict of interest.

## Author details

Priscilla Yeye Adumoah Attafuah[1*], Cecilia Eliason[1] and Ninon P. Amertil[2]

1 School of Nursing and Midwifery, University of Ghana, Legon, Ghana

2 School of Nursing and Midwifery, Valley View University, Oyibi, Ghana

*Address all correspondence to: pyaattafuah@ug.edu.gh

## References

[1] Ashirifi GD, Karikari G, Adamek ME. Prioritizing the National Aging Policy in Ghana: Critical next steps. Journal of Aging & Social Policy. 2022;**34**(1):127-144

[2] Galvin AE, Friedman DB, Hébert JR. Focus on disability-free life expectancy: Implications for health-related quality of life. Quality of Life Research. 2021;**30**(8):2187-2195

[3] Laddu D, Paluch AE, LaMonte MJ. The role of the built environment in promoting movement and physical activity across the lifespan: Implications for public health. Progress in Cardiovascular Diseases. 2021;**64**:33-40

[4] Wickramasinghe K, Mathers JC, Wopereis S, Marsman DS, Griffiths JC. From lifespan to healthspan: The role of nutrition in healthy ageing. Journal of Nutritional Science. 2020;**9**:e33

[5] Kocman D, Regen E, Phelps K, Martin G, Parker S, Gilbert T, et al. Can comprehensive geriatric assessment be delivered without the need for geriatricians? A formative evaluation in two perioperative surgical settings. Age and Ageing. 2019;**48**(5):644-649

[6] Zubair M, Chadborn NH, Gladman JR, Dening T, Gordon AL, Goodman C. Using comprehensive geriatric assessment for quality improvements in healthcare of older people in UK care homes: Protocol for realist review within Proactive Healthcare of Older People in Care Homes (PEACH) study. BMJ Open. 2017;**7**(10):e017270

[7] Kelly G, Mrengqwa L, Geffen L. "They don't care about us": Older people's experiences of primary healthcare in Cape Town, South Africa. BMC Geriatrics. 2019;**19**(1):1-4

[8] Lennaerts H, Steppe M, Munneke M, Meinders MJ, van der Steen JT, Van den Brand M, et al. Palliative care for persons with Parkinson's disease: A qualitative study on the experiences of health care professionals. BMC Palliative Care. 2019;**18**(1):1-9

[9] Arulanandem K, Jayawickramaraja PT, Hettige S, Ramanayake RP, Kisokanth G. Health care needs and services available for elders in the Batticaloa district. 2018;**34**:3-10

[10] Lum HD, Nearing K, Pimentel CB, Levy CR, Hung WW. Anywhere to anywhere: Use of telehealth to increase health care access for older, rural veterans. Public Policy & Aging Report. 2020;**30**(1):12-18

[11] Flaherty E, Bartels SJ. Addressing the community-based geriatric healthcare workforce shortage by leveraging the potential of interprofessional teams. Journal of the American Geriatrics Society. 2019;**67**(S2):S400-S408

[12] Rezaei-Shahsavarloo Z, Atashzadeh-Shoorideh F, Gobbens RJ, Ebadi A, Ghaedamini HG. The impact of interventions on management of frailty in hospitalized frail older adults: A systematic review and meta-analysis. BMC Geriatrics. 2020;**20**(1):1-7

[13] Middleton M. Orthogeriatrics and hip fracture care in the UK: Factors driving change to more integrated models of care. Geriatrics. 2018;**3**(3):55

[14] World Health Organization. Global action plan on the public health response to dementia 2017-2025. In Global action plan on the public health response to dementia 2017-2025. 2017

[15] World Health Organization, World Health Organization. Ageing, life course unit. In: WHO Global Report on Falls Prevention in Older Age. Geneva, Switzerland: World Health Organization Press; 2008

[16] Pedell S, Borda A, Keirnan A, Aimers N. Combining the digital, social and physical layer to create age-friendly cities and communities. International Journal of Environmental Research and Public Health. 2021;**18**(1):325

[17] Røsvik J, Rokstad AM. What are the needs of people with dementia in acute hospital settings, and what interventions are made to meet these needs? A systematic integrative review of the literature. BMC Health Services Research. 2020;**20**(1):1-20

[18] Tanyi PL, Pelser A. Towards an "age-friendly-hospital": Older persons' perceptions of an age-friendly hospital environment in Nigeria. Cogent Medicine. 2020;**7**(1):1853895

[19] Rodríguez Mañas L, García-Sánchez I, Hendry A, Bernabei R, Roller-Wirnsberger R, Gabrovec B, et al. Key messages for a frailty prevention and management policy in Europe from the advantage joint action consortium. The Journal of Nutrition, Health & Aging. 2018;**22**(8):892-897

[20] Bhattacharya SB, Bhattacharya RK, Turner TA. Novel model to teach health care delivery in geriatrics. Gerontology & Geriatrics Education. 2 Oct 2022;**43**(4):571-583

[21] Officer A, Schneiders ML, Wu D, Nash P, Thiyagarajan JA, Beard JR. Valuing older people: Time for a global campaign to combat ageism. Bulletin of the World Health Organization. 2016;**94**(10):710

[22] Che CC, Chong MC, Hairi NN. What influences student nurses' intention to work with older people? A cross-sectional study. International Journal of Nursing Studies. 2018;**85**:61-67

[23] Searby A, Maude P, McGrath I. The experiences of clinicians caring for older adults with dual diagnosis: An exploratory study. Issues in Mental Health Nursing. 2017;**38**(10):805-811

[24] Che CC, Chong MC, Hairi NN. What influences student nurses' intention to work with older people? A cross-sectional study. International Journal of Nursing Studies. 1 Sep 2018;**85**:61-67

[25] Alabaf Sabbaghi S, De Souza D, Sarikonda P, Keevil VL, Wallis SJ, Romero-Ortuno R. Allocating patients to geriatric medicine wards in a tertiary university hospital in England: A service evaluation of the Specialist Advice for the Frail Elderly (SAFE) team. Aging Medicine. 2018;**1**(2):120-124

[26] Banerjee J, Conroy S, Cooke MW. Quality care for older people with urgent and emergency care needs in UK emergency departments. Emergency Medicine Journal. 2013;**30**(9):699-700

[27] DesRoches C, Chang Y, Kim J, Mukunda S, Norman L, Dittus RS, et al. Who wants to work in geriatrics: Findings from a national survey of physicians and nurse practitioners. Nursing Outlook. 1 Mar 2022;**70**(2):309-314

[28] McAvoy S, Staib A, Treston G. Can a system dynamics model of the emergency department show which levers reduce bottlenecks and delays to improve access to care? Systems Research and Behavioral Science. 2021;**38**(1):61-79

[29] Cooper E, Spilsbury K, McCaughan D, Thompson C, Butterworth T, Hanratty B. Priorities for the professional development of registered nurses in nursing homes: A Delphi study. Age and Ageing. 2017;**46**(1):39-45

[30] Evans R, Larkins S, Cheffins T, Fleming R, Johnston K, Tennant M. Mapping access to health services as a strategy for planning: access to primary care for older people in regional Queensland. Australian Journal of Primary Health. 2017;**23**(2):114-122

[31] Dawud M, Kotecho MG, Adamek ME. "It is all about giving priority to older adults' needs:" Challenges of formal caregivers in two old age homes in Ethiopia. Ageing International. 2022;**47**(4):847-865

[32] Dovie DA. The status of older adult care in contemporary Ghana: A profile of some emerging issues. Frontiers in Sociology. 2019;**4**:25

[33] Brown RT, Hemati K, Riley ED, Lee CT, Ponath C, Tieu L, et al. Geriatric conditions in a population-based sample of older homeless adults. The Gerontologist. 2017;**57**(4):757-766

[34] Jeste DV, Blazer DG II, Buckwalter KC, Cassidy KL, Fishman L, Gwyther LP, et al. Age-friendly communities initiative: Public health approach to promoting successful aging. The American Journal of Geriatric Psychiatry. 2016;**24**(12):1158-1170

[35] Knowler J, Webb EO. 'Grandly designing' cohousing for older people in Australia: Overcoming the challenges. In: The Age-friendly Lens. Routledge, United Kingdom; 5 Aug 2022. pp. 136-162

[36] Luciano A, Pascale F, Polverino F, Pooley A. Measuring age-friendly housing: A framework. Sustainability. 2020;**12**(3):848

[37] Power ER. Mobility-based disadvantage in older age: Insecure housing and the risks of moving house. Ageing & Society. 2022;**42**(1):89-111

[38] Coyle MA, Chang HC, Burns P, Traynor V. Impact of interactive education on health care practitioners and older adults at risk of delirium: A literature review. Journal of Gerontological Nursing. 2018;**44**(8):41-48

[39] Crownover JG, Henrichs KA. Improving nursing student attitudes toward older adults through the use of Mask-Ed™ simulation. Journal of Gerontological Nursing. 2021;**47**(12):43-47

[40] Liu YE, Norman IJ, While AE. Nurses' attitudes towards older people and working with older patients: An explanatory model. Journal of Nursing Management. 2015;**23**(8):965-973

[41] Oliver D, Foot C, Humphries R. Making Our Health and Care Systems Fit for an Ageing Population. London: UK: King's Fund; 2014

[42] American Geriatrics Society. American Geriatrics Society (AGS) policy brief: COVID-19 and assisted living facilities. Journal of the American Geriatrics Society. 2020;**68**(6):1131-1135

[43] Mezey M, Kobayashi M, Grossman S, Firpo A, Fulmer T, Mitty E. Nurses improving care to health system elders (NICHE): Implementation of best practice models. JONA: The Journal of Nursing Administration. 2004;**34**(10):451-457

Chapter 12

# The Effect of Chromotherapy on Decreased Blood Pressure during Sleep in Hypertension Patients in Kupang, Indonesia

*Serly Sani Mahoklory and Ferdinandus Suban Hoda*

## Abstract

Various efforts to prevent the increasing prevalence of deaths due to hypertension continue to be developed, including alternative medicine systems (CAMS). One of the alternative treatment methods recommended by the world, easy, cheap, and efficient is chromotherapy or light therapy. The purpose of this study was to look at the influence of chromotherapy in lowering blood pressure during sleep in hypertension sufferers. The research method used is quasy experiment with the design of one group pre- and posttest with a control group design. Sampling techniques are carried out using purposive sampling with the number of 120 respondents. The results of this study have proven that chromotherapy has a tremendous effect in lowering blood pressure by 10–30 mmHg during sleep 15–35 minutes by utilizing the blue and green spectrum that affects the work of the sympathetic and parasympathetic nerves so as to provide elements of relaxation and lower blood pressure. The pretest result of the treatment group obtained a mean from 172/96 to 158/93 mmHg, which showed a decrease while in the control group, there was no significant change with mean values of 166/96 and 166/97 mmHg.

**Keywords:** chromotherapy, electromagnetic radiation, hypertension, blood pressure, Indonesia

## 1. Introduction

The prevalence of hypertension is increasing every year and is a leading cause of 13% global mortality. This condition is projected to increase by up to 30% of global mortality in 2025 [1]. Most of the hypertension-related-death in the world occurs in low- and-middle-income countries (31,5%) compared to high-income countries (28.5%) [2]. Indonesia is one of the middle-income countries whose prevalence of hypertension has increased from 25.8% in 2013 to 34.1% in 2018 [3]. The national prevalence for coronary heart disease is 1.5%, and the highest prevalence is in the East Nusa Tenggara (NTT) province at 4.4%.

Pharmacological treatment is the main choice for lowering blood pressure. However, along with the development of technology, non-pharmacological treatment has become one of the recommended alternative treatments for hypertension treatment based on evidence-based practice. The use of complementary therapies and alternative medicine (CAM) continues to grow and the majority of people with hypertension. This is because the side effects produced are lower than that of pharmacological treatment. The relatively cheaper cost and the same effectiveness are indicators of the use of complementary and alternative therapies in the treatment of hypertension. One of the therapies that can be used to lower blood pressure in people with hypertension is chromotherapy [4–6].

Chromotherapy or color therapy is a complementary alternative treatment recommended globally, utilizing electromagnetic radiation and several color frequencies to affect human neurohormonal pathways. With this mechanism, chromotherapy can cure various diseases [7–9]. The color effects work by intervening in the action of the sympathetic and parasympathetic nerves. Color therapy provides a relaxation element, reducing an individual's anxiety level [10]. The use of green and blue lights in chromotherapy help reduce stress levels and lower blood pressure in patients with hypertension *via* epinephrine hormone stimulation. This study aimed to determine the effectiveness of chromotherapy in blood pressure in hypertension patients in Oesapa Primary Health Care Center (Puskesmas). It can be hypothesized that chromotherapy can significantly reduce lower blood pressure in patients with hypertension.

## 2. Methods

This is a quasi-experimental study with one group pre and posttest with one control group design. The treatment group was given chromotherapy treatment, while the control group was not. The blood pressure was measured at baseline (pretest) and after the treatment was performed (posttest) for both groups [11, 12]. A total of 120 hypertension patients participated in this study. The participants were divided equally into two groups; 60 participants in the treatment group and another 60 participants in the control group. Data were analyzed using Mann–Whitney U test to determine any difference between the pre and posttest scores for each group. The level of significance was determined at $p$-value <0.05. Statistical analysis was performed using IBM SPSS™ software.

This study incorporates a combination of green and blue LED lights. The intervention was conducted in a closed room using a 50 cm light transmission device, and then hung or placed 210 cm above the participant's body and left for 15–35 minutes. Participants were requested to relax and close their eyes during the intervention. After the intervention, the respondent's blood pressure was measured again.

## 3. Results

### 3.1 General data

See **Table 1**

| Characteristic | Category | Groups | | | | p-value |
|---|---|---|---|---|---|---|
| | | Intervention | | Control | | |
| | | n | % | N | % | |
| Gender | Male | 28 | 46,7 | 30 | 50 | 0,592 |
| | Female | 32 | 53,3 | 30 | 50 | |
| Total | | 60 | 100 | 60 | 100 | |
| Age | 40–45 | 18 | 30 | 17 | 28,3 | 0,201 |
| | 46–50 | 29 | 48,3 | 29 | 48,3 | |
| | 51–55 | 13 | 21,7 | 14 | 23,3 | |
| Total | | 60 | 100 | 60 | 100 | |
| Level of Education | Elementary School | 3 | 5 | 3 | 5 | |
| | Junior High School | 4 | 6,7 | 8 | 13,3 | |
| | Senior High School | 25 | 41,7 | 22 | 36,7 | |
| | Bachelor | 26 | 43,3 | 26 | 43,3 | |
| | Master - Graduate | 2 | 3,3 | 1 | 1,7 | |
| Total | | 60 | 100 | 60 | 100 | |

*Source: Primary Data 2020*

**Table 1.**
*Characteristics of participants based on gender, age, and education level of the working area of Oesapa primary health care Center Kupang.*

| Variables | Category | Pretest | | Posttest | |
|---|---|---|---|---|---|
| Blood Pressure | Intervention | F | % | F | % |
| | Normal | 0 | 0 | | 0 |
| | Prehypertension | 0 | 0 | 1 | 1,7 |
| | Stage 1 Hypertension | 13 | 21,7 | 38 | 63,3 |
| | Stage 2 Hypertension | 45 | 75 | 21 | 35 |
| | Isolated Systolic Hypertension | 2 | 3,3 | 0 | 0 |
| | Total | 60 | 100% | 60 | 100% |
| | **Control** | | | | |
| | Normal | 0 | 0 | 0 | 0 |
| | Prehypertension | 3 | 5 | 0 | 0 |
| | Stage 1 Hypertension | 29 | 48,3 | 19 | 32,7 |
| | Stage 2 Hypertension | 27 | 45 | 39 | 65 |
| | Isolated Systolic Hypertension | 1 | 1,7 | 2 | 3,3 |
| | Total | 60 | 100% | 60 | 100 |

*Source: Primary Data 2020.*

**Table 2.**
*Distribution blood pressure of hypertension of the working area of Oesapa primary health care Center Kupang.*

| Resp | Blood Pressure Intervention Groups | | Blood Pressure Control Groups | |
|---|---|---|---|---|
| | Pretest | Posttest | Pretest | Posttest |
| 1 | 160/100 | 155/100 | 170/100 | 170/100 |
| 2 | 150/100 | 140/90 | 190/110 | 190/100 |
| 3 | 140/90 | 135/90 | 180/100 | 160/100 |
| 4 | 140/90 | 140/90 | 160/100 | 160/105 |
| 5 | 150/100 | 145/100 | 210/110 | 210/120 |
| 6 | 180/90 | 175/90 | 180/90 | 180/100 |
| 7 | 170/100 | 170/90 | 200/120 | 200/110 |
| 8 | 180/110 | 180/100 | 150/100 | 150/100 |
| 9 | 210/100 | 200/100 | 140/100 | 140/100 |
| 10 | 170/110 | 170/115 | 180/110 | 180/110 |
| 11 | 180/100 | 180/90 | 190/120 | 190/100 |
| 12 | 180/110 | 180/90 | 140/90 | 140/100 |
| 13 | 150/90 | 145/90 | 140/80 | 140/90 |
| 14 | 150/80 | 145/80 | 160/100 | 165/100 |
| 15 | 180/100 | 170/100 | 145/90 | 145/90 |
| 16 | 160/90 | 150/90 | 150/80 | 160/90 |
| 17 | 170/100 | 160/95 | 180/100 | 180/90 |
| 18 | 150/80 | 150/80 | 160/80 | 190/100 |
| 19 | 180/90 | 150/90 | 150/90 | 150/90 |
| 20 | 160/100 | 160/100 | 200/120 | 200/100 |
| 21 | 190/90 | 175/90 | 190/110 | 180/100 |
| 22 | 180/100 | 160/90 | 190/100 | 190/100 |
| 23 | 170/90 | 170/90 | 180/90 | 180/100 |
| 24 | 180/110 | 180/100 | 160/90 | 150/90 |
| 25 | 180/110 | 170/110 | 160/100 | 170/100 |
| 26 | 160/90 | 150/90 | 160/90 | 170/100 |
| 27 | 170/90 | 160/90 | 150/80 | 150/90 |
| 28 | 160/90 | 150/90 | 170/110 | 170/100 |
| 29 | 180/90 | 155/90 | 160/90 | 160/90 |
| 30 | 180/90 | 170/90 | 150/100 | 160/90 |
| 31 | 190/90 | 160/80 | 180/90 | 170/100 |
| 32 | 180/100 | 155/90 | 150/90 | 140/90 |
| 33 | 170/100 | 140/90 | 140/90 | 150/90 |
| 34 | 170/100 | 150/90 | 170/90 | 180/100 |
| 35 | 160/100 | 150/90 | 180/100 | 180/100 |
| 36 | 170/100 | 160/90 | 180/90 | 170/100 |
| 37 | 180/100 | 150/100 | 160/90 | 170/100 |

| Resp | Blood Pressure Intervention Groups | | Blood Pressure Control Groups | |
|---|---|---|---|---|
| | Pretest | Posttest | Pretest | Posttest |
| 38 | 160/90 | 150/100 | 160/100 | 160/100 |
| 39 | 170/100 | 170/100 | 150/100 | 150/100 |
| 40 | 180/100 | 160/90 | 170/90 | 160/100 |
| 41 | 180/90 | 165/90 | 180/90 | 180/90 |
| 42 | 170/100 | 150/100 | 150/100 | 150/100 |
| 43 | 180/100 | 170/100 | 150/105 | 150/105 |
| 44 | 170/80 | 155/90 | 150/100 | 150/90 |
| 45 | 160/100 | 160/100 | 170/90 | 170/80 |
| 46 | 180/100 | 160/90 | 180/100 | 180/90 |
| 47 | 190/100 | 160/80 | 180/90 | 170/90 |
| 48 | 190/90 | 140/90 | 180/100 | 180/100 |
| 49 | 180/100 | 140/100 | 160/100 | 150/100 |
| 50 | 170/100 | 140/100 | 160/90 | 170/100 |
| 51 | 160/90 | 150/80 | 150/90 | 160/100 |
| 52 | 170/100 | 150/100 | 180/90 | 170/100 |
| 53 | 170/100 | 140/100 | 160/90 | 150/100 |
| 54 | 180/80 | 165/90 | 160/90 | 150/90 |
| 55 | 180/100 | 160/90 | 180/80 | 180/80 |
| 56 | 190/80 | 180/100 | 160/80 | 150/90 |
| 57 | 200/90 | 150/90 | 150/90 | 160/80 |
| 58 | 170/100 | 150/90 | 150/100 | 150/105 |
| 59 | 170/80 | 140/80 | 150/90 | 160/100 |
| 60 | 160/100 | 150/90 | 160/100 | 160/100 |
| **Rata-rata** | **172/96** | **168/93** | **166/96** | **166/97** |

*Sumber: Data Primer 2020.*

**Table 3.**
*Distribution of blood pressure pre and post intervention and control groups of working area of Oesapa primary health care Center Kupang.*

## 3.2 Specific data

The pretest was performed at baseline to understand the respondent's initial blood pressure before chromotherapy treatment was given.

**Table 2** shows that chromotherapy treatment can reduce blood pressure. After receiving chromotherapy treatment and the blood pressure was reevaluated, the blood pressure had improved to a level I hypertension (63.3%). On the contrary, there was no significant decrease in blood pressure for the control group; level I hypertension (48.3%) at the pretest and increased to level II hypertension (65%) at posttest.

**Table 3** shows the results of the blood pressure of the intervention and control groups before participating in chromotherapy did not experience a

| Tekanan Darah | Control | Mean | SD | Min-Max | p-value |
|---|---|---|---|---|---|
| Before intervention chromotherapy | intervention (n = 60) | 69,81 | 0,469 | 3–5 | 0,001 |
| | Control (n = 60) | 51,19 | 0,596 | 2–5 | |
| After intervention chromotherapy | intervention (n = 60) | 49,99 | 0,510 | 2–4 | 0,000 |
| | Control (n = 60) | 71,01 | 0,524 | 3–5 | |

*Sumber: Data Primer 2020.*

**Table 4.**
*Analisis Beda mean tingkat Stres kelompok perlakuan dan kontrol.*

significant difference, namely the mean blood pressure of the treatment group was 172/96 mmHg and the group 166/96 mmHg. Meanwhile, after participating in chromotherapy, there was a decrease in the average blood pressure of the intervention group, namely 168/93 mmHg and the control group did not experience a decrease in blood pressure, namely 166/97 mmHg. So the average decrease in blood pressure after following chromotherapy is 10–14 mmHg.

**Table 4** shows the mean blood pressure in the treatment group before the intervention was 69.81, while the blood pressure in the control group was 51.19. The results of further tests using the Mann–Whitney U Test showed no significant difference in blood pressure scores of hypertensive patients between the treatment and control groups before being given chromotherapy. After treatment, blood pressure in the treatment group decreased significantly compared to the control group (p = 0.000) and the mean blood pressure score in the treatment group decreased to 49.99, while the control group did not experience a decrease in blood pressure and tended to experience an increase in blood pressure, namely 71.01.

## 4. Discussion

This quasi-experimental study is one of the initial studies exploring the effects of color therapy on the stress levels of hypertension patients. In chromotherapy, a color is a form of electromagnetic energy and visible light. When it enters the retina's photoreceptors, it will be translated as a color that stimulates the pituitary and pineal glands to produce hormones, such as serotonin and endorphin. These hormones are secreted as a response to light to maintain psychological health, balancing mood, feelings, and behavior [13, 14]. This study uses a green and blue light that specifically has been proven to reduce blood pressure by utilizing reflected green and blue light. Combining these colors with light could selectively repair damaged cells and provide the healing energy needed [15–17].

A report by Gul et al. (2016) reinforced the result of this study, which exhibits both mild and severe stress in both groups during pretest. After the treatment group received chromotherapy treatment, there was a reduction in blood pressure score up to 10–14 mmHg with a p-value of 0.000. This means that there was a change in the initial blood pressure. Results indicated a decline of the mean blood pressure in the treatment group from 172/96 mmHg during pretest, to 158/93 during posttest. It suggests a drop of 10–14 mmHg. In the meantime, the control group did not record any significant change with a mean blood pressure of 166/96 mmHg during pretest and 166/97 during posttest. Still, a reduction in blood pressure can also be explained by categories of hypertension. Before the treatment, most of the participants in the treatment group were at level II hypertension (75%). Posttest measurement after the chromotherapy treatment displayed an improvement with 63.3% of the participants recording level I hypertension. On the other hand, no significant change was found. Most of the participants in the control group recorded level I hypertension during pretest (48.3%) and level II hypertension in posttest (65%).

The mechanism of chromotherapy in the body utilize electromagnetic radiation and different color frequency by affecting the human neurohormonal system from the sympathetic and parasympathetic nerves, thus giving it a relaxation effect, which can reduce anxiety [10]. Also, chromotherapy can heal various illnesses by utilizing seven color lights, for example, yellow for gastric ulcer, a combination of red and blue for skin infections, etc. [15]. The effect of color and light from chromotherapy can be used as an easy, inexpensive alternative nonpharmacologic treatment with minimum risk of side effects.

This study has several limitations, including a relatively small sample size (120 participants) with a short time span to measure stress level and blood pressure, which was within the three times intervention. However, this study has shown the efficacy of chromotherapy using green and blue lights after accounting for several biases during the study.

## 5. Nursing implication

Nurses can implement chromotherapy in their environment as an alternative treatment aside from pharmacologic medication, which is a new innovation in complementary therapy. Also, this study adds to the nursing reference regarding the efficacy of color therapy in reducing stress and lowering blood pressure in hypertension patients. It is recommended for forthcoming studies to increase the sample size and lengthen the timespan of the measurement by also including other color lights.

## 6. Conclusion

Chromotherapy with a combination of green and blue lights is proven to be effective to stimulate the pituitary and pineal glands to produce hormones such as serotonin and endorphin, thus maintaining psychological health, balancing mood, feelings, repairing impaired cells, and providing healing energy that the body needs. Therefore, this study recommends the use of chromotherapy to reduce stress and lower blood pressure for hypertension patients.

## Author details

Serly Sani Mahoklory* and Ferdinandus Suban Hoda
STIKes Maranatha Kupang, Indonesia

*Address all correspondence to: sani.mahoklory04@gmail.com

## References

[1] Chowdhury MZI, Rahman M, Akter T, Akhter T, Ahmed A, Shovon MA, et al. Hypertension prevalence and its trend in Bangladesh: Evidence from a systematic review and meta-analysis. Clinical Hypertension. 2020;**26**(1). DOI: 10.1186/s40885-020-00143-1

[2] Mills KT, Bundy JD, Kelly TN, Reed JE, Kearney PM, Reynolds K, et al. Global disparities of hypertension prevalence and control. Circulation. 2016;**134**(6):441-450. DOI: 10.1161/CIRCULATIONAHA.115.018912

[3] Basic Health Survey. RISKESDAS MAIN RESULT. 2018

[4] World Health Organization. Depression [Internet]. 2012 [cited 4 November 2015]. Available from: http://www.who.int/ mental_health/management/depression/en/

[5] Id MJG, Tardif H, Id MB, Tonkin A, Arnold A. Hypertension prevalence in patients attending tertiary pain management services, a registry-based Australian cohort study. 1-19. 2020

[6] Khalifeh AH. The effect of chronotherapy on depressive symptoms: Evidence-based practice. Saudi Medical Journal. 2017;**38**(5):457-464. DOI: 10.15537/smj.2017.5.18062

[7] Jones R. 基因的改变NIH public access. Bone. 2014;**23**(1):1-7. DOI: 10.1016/j.comppsych.2010.07.002.Illness

[8] Lam RW, Kennedy SH, Grigoriadis S, McIntyre RS, Milev R, Ramasubbu R, et al. Canadian network for mood and anxiety treatments (CANMAT) clinical guidelines for the management of major depressive disorder in adults. III. Pharmacotherapy. Journal of Affective Disorders. 2009;**117**(SUPPL. 1):S26-S43. DOI: 10.1016/j.jad.2009.06.041

[9] Gul S, Nadeem RK, Aslam A. Chromo therapy- an effective treatment option or just a myth? Critical Analysis on the Effectiveness of Chromo therapy. 2015;**1**(2):62-70

[10] Zola N, Fadli RP, Ifdil I. Chromotherapy to Reducing Stress. 2018. DOI: 10.31219/osf.io/dvwer

[11] Sugiyono. Educational Research Methods with Quantitative Approaches, Qualitative, and R & D. Bandung: Alfabeta; 2013

[12] Nursalam. Nursing Research Methodology: A Practical Approach. Ed 3 ed. Jakarta: Salemba Medika; 2013

[13] Hermida RC, Ayala DE, Fernández JR, Mojón A. Hypertension: New perspective on its definition and clinical management by bedtime therapy substantially reduces cardiovascular disease risk. 2017. DOI: 10.1111/eci.12909

[14] Of AB, Dults OLA, Xperimental AQU, et al. Effects of chromotherapy on the cognitive age study explore. 2019;**15**(3):191-197. DOI: 10.1016/j.explore.2019.01.002

[15] National Center for Complementary and Alternative Medicine. Complementary, Alternative, or Integrative Health: What's In a Name? [Internet]. [Updated 2008; cited 2015 November 3]. Available from: http://nccam.nih.gov/health/whatiscam

[16] Yousuf ST, Rafiq HM, Ismail I, Rabab S. Complementary therapies in medicine the mechanistic basis of chromotherapy: Current

knowledge and future perspectives. Complementary Therapies in Medicine. 2019;**46**(August):217-222. DOI: 10.1016/j.ctim.2019.08.025

[17] Sajatovic M, Levin J, Fuentes-Casiano E, Cassidy KA, Tatsuoka C, Jenkins JH. Illness Experience and Reasons for nonadherence among individuals with bipolar disorder who are poorly adherent with medication. Comprehensive Psychiatry. 2011;**52**(3):280-287. DOI: 10.1016/j.comppsych.2010.07.002

Chapter 13

# Nurses Work System Optimization: Macroergonomics Perspective

*Ehsan Garosi*


## Abstract

The hospital work system as a complex sociotechnical system has been an interesting research environment for human factor/ergonomic researchers. In this chapter dimensions of nurses' work system elements were presented and Macroergonomics approaches were pointed out to optimize the interaction between nurses and other system elements. From Macroergonomics perspectives, human factor researchers would be able to identify and categorize health and performance issues through a systematic approach. Researchers are believed that this approach was not shown positive results initially, therefore a low-hanging fruit strategy is recommended. Decomposing work system elements is a potential opportunity to track the balance in the hospital nurse work system by considering these elements for redesigning work systems and applying appropriate interventions.


**Keywords:** nurses, ergonomics, human factor, design, performance

## 1. Introduction

> *To reap what we sowed, "we should start with the low-hanging fruits"*
>
> *(Michael Porter in 1980).*

Hospital work system as a complex sociotechnical system has been an interesting research environment for the human factor/ergonomic researchers. Among health care workers, nurses have always been considered to be a special group because of the significant physical and mental demands they face at work. Nursing is a physically and psychologically demanding profession with a high prevalence of musculoskeletal disorders (MSDs) as indicated in several studies [1–5]. MSDs are also often cited as the reason for sickness-related absences and the high turnover of nurses [6, 7].

Nurses' working conditions usually differ across countries, regions, and hospitals [8, 9]. These differences are attributed mainly to the provision of instruments and the quality of process management in hospitals. For instance, nurses whom working in intensive care units may experiences higher stress levels and more health disorders compared with other wards [10].

There are many factors that can influence on nurses working conditions [11]. Therefore, seeking and attenuating these risk factors (risk factors that affect on nurses' health and working performance) requires a systematic and comprehensive

| Authors | Title | Conclusion |
|---|---|---|
| Carayon et al., [11] | Macroergonomics in Healthcare Quality and Patient Safety | Study of job stress and burnout, workload, interruptions, patient-centered care, health IT and medical devices, violations, and care coordination provide examples of Macroergonomics contributions to healthcare quality and patient safety. Macroergonomics models of healthcare quality and patient safety are well-accepted by the healthcare community Hence, the potential impact of Macroergonomics on refining care processes and patient outcomes is important. |
| Punnett et al., [16] | Participatory Ergonomics as a Model for Integrated Programs to Prevent Chronic Disease | Participatory ergonomics is pertinent to workplace health promotion (WHP) because (1) psychosocial stress backs to individual health behaviors as well as chronic diseases; (2) job stress cannot be spoken without employee envelopment in hazard identification and solutions; (3) the interaction of multiple levels within an organization requires consideration to necessities and limitations at all levels. |
| Guimarães et al., [17] | Worker evaluation of a Macroergonomics intervention in a Brazilian footwear company | This study showed that problems and resolutions can be recognized through participatory ergonomics, that it is easier to include workers than the managerial staff, and that a Macroergonomics intervention, mainly focusing on work organization, led to positive employees, health and production results, despite management's opposition to changes multiskilling and teamwork were the foremost changes promoted to increase and improve work and make it more flexible. |
| Adelt et al., [18] | Governance of complex systems: results of a sociological simulation experiment | Practitioner can have oriented into functioning of complex systems and acquire how to well manage them. Moreover, they can ever measure the performance. |
| Murphy et al., [19] | The next generation of Macroergonomics: Integrating safety climate | Investigating safety climate with concerns to a systems method is a zone of research that is growing. Whereas safety climate is a principal indicator of safety, it is used more often to measure the level of general safety in an organization and not to determine where safety problems happen. Hence, the concept needs to be complemented with a Macroergonomics approach to design work systems accordingly that we can recognize specific human-technology organization interfaces within an organization that negatively and positively affect the safety consciousness of workers' in that organization. |
| Clack et al., [20] | low-hanging fruit for human factors design in infection prevention still too high to reach? | In the progressively sophisticated and complex health care system, future infection prevention success on not only moving from standard operating procedures to engineered solutions but also how well we govern trans-institutional complexity. |
| Karsh et al., [21] | Crossing levels in systems ergonomics: A framework to support 'Macroergonomics' inquiry | "Macroergonomics is defined as an open systems approach to human factors and ergonomics (HFE) theory and research whereby the connection between variables in at least two different system levels is studied, and where the dependent variables are human factors and ergonomic constructs." |
| Carayon et al., [22] | Human factors systems approach to healthcare quality and patient safety | Harmonizing the work system and boosting the dynamic and adaptive role of workers are important principles for improving healthcare quality and patient safety. |
| Carayon et al., [22] | Healthcare workers' perceptions of lean: A context-sensitive, mixed methods study in three Swedish hospitals | Hospital workers' perceptions of lean differ by hospital, unit, and role study approves that background problems and sheds some light on how specific lean intervention plans in definite settings influence employees' primary perceptions of lean. |

| Authors | Title | Conclusion |
|---|---|---|
| Village et al., [23] | design for human factors (DfHF): a grounded theory for integrating human factors into production design processes | The DfHF grounded theory delivers empirical evidence that fills a gap by showing 'how' HF characteristics can be combined into the production design process to increase worker performance and well-being |
| Waterson et al., [24] | Defining the methodological challenges and opportunities for an effective science of sociotechnical systems and safety | This article is described sociotechnical systems theory STS methods for workplace safety, as well as outlining a set of six case studies covering the application of these methods to a range of safety contexts |
| Salas et al., [25] | Measuring Team Cohesion: Observations from the Science | "However long considered a key contributor to team success, cohesion is perhaps more important than ever. As organizations continue to seek competitive advantage, teams are increasingly looked to in the hopes of facilitating knowledge, morale, and creativity." |
| Kleiner et al., [26] | Sociotechnical attributes of safe and unsafe work systems | Sociotechnical methodologies to workplace safety highlight the critical importance of design through the sociotechnical field. Given the dramatic progress in complexity of everyday work systems, sociotechnical systems thinking be able to possibly most helpfully be assumed of as providing a set of constructs, objectives and methods to support vital efforts to joint optimization of system element and interactions. |
| Realyvásquez et al., [27] | Structural Model for the Effects of Environmental Elements on the Psychological Characteristics and Performance of the Employees of Manufacturing Systems | The Macroergonomics compatibility of environmental elements shows a important straight effects on participant psychological characteristics and also direct or indirect effects on the workers' performance. |
| Bolis and Sznelwar, [28] | A case study of the implementation of an ergonomics improvement committee in a Brazilian Hospital Challenges and benefits | The findings of this study shows that good consequences require autonomy and support from management, and the adoption of effective methods to increase and legitimize the development committee's life. |
| Steege and Dykstra, [29] | A Macroergonomics perspective on fatigue and coping in the hospital nurse work system | "A Macroergonomics approach is valuable for understanding complexities of work system barriers and facilitators to fatigue and coping." |
| Azadeh et al., [30] | Optimization of healthcare supply chain in context of macro-ergonomics factors by a unique mathematical programming approach | This is the first study for Macroergonomics optimization of healthcare supply chain. This technique can examine the influence of Macroergonomics factors on supply chain management in healthcare environment. Correspondingly, this technique ranks the pertinent performance efficiencies of each healthcare supply chain. This study by using proposed method, indicates on "teamwork" topic as is a well-known topic in Macroergonomics. Furthermore, this study would help managers to detect the areas of faults in their supply chain management system and fixed them by improvement target plan for the related supply chain management system in healthcare environments. |

| Authors | Title | Conclusion |
|---|---|---|
| Yang and Asan, [31] | Designing patient-facing health information technologies for the outpatient settings: a literature review | The designs of patient-facing health information technologies (HITs) in outpatient sites are likely by easing the doctor-patient communication and patient engagement. Conversely, their effectiveness and usefulness need to be additional assessment and improved from a systems viewpoint. |
| Meshkati et al., [32] | People-Technology-Ecosystem Integration: A Framework to Ensure Regional Interoperability for Safety, Sustainability, and Resilience of Interdependent Energy, Water, and Seafood Sources in the (Persian) Gulf | Based on the emerging realities in the Gulf region, it is concluded that without systematic approach concerning to interdependencies of water and energy sources, sustainability will be just a short-lived dream and success will be a disappearing mirage for millions of people that live in this area. |
| Thatcher and Yeow, [33] | A sustainable system of systems approach: a new HFE paradigm | This study present a sustainable system of systems model that joins ideas from the ecological sciences, particularly a nested order of systems and a hierarchical time aspect. |
| Holden et al., [34] | Macroergonomic Factors in the Patient Work System: Examining the Context of Patients with Chronic Illness | After present 3 relevant case findings: proved that not only the importance of setting for patients' health-related activities but also specific factors to study in future research, design, and policy efforts. |
| Coelho et al., [35] | Psychosocial and ergonomic survey of office and field jobs in a utility company | For most psychosocial aspects, the organizational design and management system in place and the overall cultural environment in which it works, create a much robust and more critical impact than job-specific factors. |
| Murphy et al., [36] | A sociotechnical systems approach to enhance safety climate in the trucking industry: Development of a methodology | Tis study proposed a mythology that can be used as a way to recognize gaps in the specific work system, and this data can be used to design interventions to change the safety climate, and finally the culture, of an organization in due to reduce negative safety consequences. |
| Murphy et al., [37] | A sociotechnical systems approach to enhance safety climate in the trucking industry: Results of an in-depth investigation | The overall goal of this study was to generate a methodology, based on a systems approach that could be used to evaluate an organizational work system as an assessment tool. The findings of this study comprised 19 themes that affect on safety. These themes fluctuated from balancing work and family-personal time, the firm's strategy vs. practice, respecting the job of the driver, and active listening and meaningful feedback. The most imperative themes were related to the workers internal environment. |
| Thatcher et al., [38] | State of Science: ergonomics and global issues | This article is showed what has been achieved by the ergonomics profession in relation to the global challenges raised by Moray's 1993 keynote address to the International Ergonomics Association. |

**Table 1.**
*Published articles concern to macroergonomic approaches.*

approach. To deal with and overcome on such ergonomic issues in the complex sociotechnical system, macro ergonomic approaches always have been shown positive and applicable [11].

### 1.1 Macroergonomic approaches as a solution

As the new millennium unfolds, there is significant evidence that the complexity of organizations is increasing and with this consistent growth comes new considerations for designing, implementing and maintaining work systems. In order to manage this growing complexity and to achieve desired outcomes, in these contexts, numerous approaches have been proposed [12]. Macroergonomics, a sub-discipline of ergonomics, has been a practical response to this growing need and with embracing this innate complexity it aims to improve performance and well-being in work systems [13].

Viewing under the Macroergonomics glasses, enables human factor researchers to identify and categorize health and performance issues through a systematic approach. In this vein, it would be helpful for identifying such factors by taking into account all components of the work system [14]. For instance, Garosi et al., used this approaches to identify influencing factors on nurses workability [15].

Lets back on Michael Porter in 1980 quotation about "piking low hanging fruits" as indicated by H. W. Hendrick and B. Kleiner [14]. This quotation is indicates on doing micro accessible intervention and then performing the macro intervention. Macroergonomics approaches help researcher to find, which work system elements are accessible and can be manipulate at first.

During this book chapter, we do a review on some studies affirmed macroergonomics approaches in similar health scope system and then we decomposed nurses work system elements with focus on their workability using the Systems Engineering Initiative for Patient Safety (SEIPS). Next, relative recommendations were provided to optimize interaction between nurses and work system element.

### 1.2 Published articles in domain of Macroergonomics

Studies on the level of Macroergonomics were searched over Google Scholar, PubMed, and Science Direct from 2013-2018. The search was conducted using such keywords including: "(Macroergonomics OR Macro-ergonomics)" The inclusion criteria were the article published in English, and all type of study (interventional or questionnaire). The database search showed 72 articles, out of which 40 were excluded because of duplication, repetition and article publication date. Among the remaining articles, a further 7 were removed due to the irrelevant subject. Finally,25 articles were left and selected for extracting the kay-pints. **Table 1** shows the article in order of publication date.

## 2. Decomposing nurses work system elements

According to the Systems Engineering Initiative for Patient Safety (SEIPS) elements of a work system comprises five components including environment, person, tools and technology, task, and organization, and their interplay determines (the processes), how care is managed and provided to patients leading to desired or undesired outcomes [39]. Following, partial results of a study [15] is presented to emphasize on SEIPS model as a framework for decomposing influencing factors on the nurse's workability.

### 2.1 Environmental elements

- The environmental elements are included:
- Layout of work space
- Work space dimensions (ingress and egress)
- Illumination
- Noise and Vibration
- Ventilation and temperature stress
- Esthetics of the workspace design (Furniture design)

Environmental conditions may interfere with nurse's task. Due to lack of space, people may work in inappropriate postures and poor lighting conditions, which can increase the risk of musculoskeletal disorders [29].

For better perception in work space, applying ornamental artificial flowers and color variations as features for motivating are recommended. However optimal design of the work environment increases the satisfaction of nurses and consequently lead to positive performance results [40].

### 2.2 Person- related factors (nurses)

- Demographic characteristics
- Ethnicity
- Working experience
- Self-esteem
- Second job

Many studies have examined the relationship between demographic characteristics, ethnicity, and diseases to the nurses work ability. For instance, high body mass index had an inverse relationship with work ability [41]. Generally, as BMI crosses over 25, the working ability of nurses decreased by 2.2 points [42]. Moreover, many studies have showed the relationship between age and work ability. Second job or worked simultaneously in two or more hospitals put nurses under more physical and mental stress, fatigue [43, 44].

### 2.3 Factors related to tools and technology

Usability of the tools and technology are reported as an important factor, which could increase satisfaction and work ability. In addition, some other factors such as equipment precision (calibration), applicability, equipment safety, computerization are reported important contributors to the nurses work ability [15]. Correspondingly, availability of equipment, proper functioning and effectiveness of tools were identified as measures to prevent nursing fatigue. Moreover, it is reported that electronic reporting and high level technology based tools may prevents nurses fatigue [29]. In this way Samadi and Golmohammadi, showed that there was a negative relationship between work ability and fatigue [45]. It is quit clear that usability of devises are important in every similar sociotechnical systems. Therefore, Lacking usability leading to fatigue and increases the risk of musculoskeletal disorders in nursing job [46]. For instance, a nurses quotation from a qualitative study is considerable “although computers and technology are much quicker and more comfortable to use, in some cases these computers and automation software are so problematic and time wasting, that we decide to do tasks manually” [15].

### 2.4 Task-related factors

Task-related factors are factors related to the nature of nursing tasks. The most important factors Identified included:

- High mental and physical demanding tasks
- Workload
- Repetitive tasks
- work cycle time/rest
- Work pace

Nursing job stressors such as inappropriate expectations from co-workers, time constraints, response to patient families are reported as other nurses job related factors that have negative effect on nursing work ability [45].

### 2.5 Organization elements

Danesh et al., 2020 reported that are more effective factor on the nurses work ability [15]. These factors included:

- Supervisor support
- Teamwork
- Staffing work regulation
- Salary and organizational policies
- Participation
- Job involvement

Quality supervisors support was reported among the most important predictors of nurses work ability. In a study by Gharibi et al. [47], which was conducted among a number of employees of different sectors, including industry, bank, and hospital, there was a straight relationship between supervisors support and work ability. Moreover, a strong correlation between supervisor support and work ability was reported [48]. Teamwork and support of colleagues are among other effective factors that influence on nurses work ability. Working under the supervision and in an efficient team and fairly performing tasks, there will be lower fatigue and team performance will be increase [49]. Shift work schedule is a factor that can affect circadian rhythm as, Safari et al. Safari et al. showed a significant relationship between work ability and work shift [50]. Other studies emphasized the role of shift work on nursing work ability, with nurses who had more than 8 hours of work shift were more likely to suffer burnout [51].

Salary and wage are factors that directly related to motivation and work ability. Under Herzberg's two-factor model, incomes and paybacks are "health" factors, which, if not sufficient, result in dissatisfaction and eventually stress and adverse outcomes [52].

## 3. Conclusions

Optimizing nurses' work system requires a holistic approach and the Macroergonomics approach could be helpful in this way. Under Macroergonomics perspectives, human factor researchers would be able to identify and categorize health and performance issues through a systematic approach. Researchers are believed that this approach was not shown positive results initially, therefore a low-hanging fruit strategy is recommended. Decomposing work system elements is a potential opportunity to track the balance in the hospital nurse work system by considering these elements for redesigning work systems and applying appropriate interventions.

## Author details

Ehsan Garosi
Department of Ergonomics, School of Public Health, Iran University of Medical Sciences, Iran

*Address all correspondence to: eh.garosi@gmail.com

## References

[1] Choobineh A, Movahed M, Tabatabaie SH, Kumashiro M. Perceived demands and musculoskeletal disorders in operating room nurses of shiraz city hospitals. Industrial Health. 2010;**48**:74-84

[2] Magnago TSBDS, Lisboa MTL, Griep RH, Kirchhof ALC, Guido LDA. Psychosocial aspects of work and musculoskeletal disorders in nursing workers. Revista Latino-Americana de Enfermagem. 2010;**18**:429-435

[3] Menzel NN. Psychosocial factors in musculoskeletal disorders. Critical Care Nursing Clinics of North America. 2007;**19**:145-153

[4] Smith DR, Mihashi M, Adachi Y, Koga H, Ishitake T. A detailed analysis of musculoskeletal disorder risk factors among Japanese nurses. Journal of Safety Research. 2006;**37**:195-200

[5] Smith DR, Sato M, Miyajima T, Mizutani T, Yamagata Z. Musculoskeletal disorders self-reported by female nursing students in Central Japan: A complete cross-sectional survey. International Journal of Nursing Studies. 2003;**40**:725-729

[6] Blekesaune M, Solem PE. Working conditions and early retirement a prospective study of retirement behavior. Research on Aging. 2005;**27**:3-30

[7] Menzel NN. Underreporting of musculoskeletal disorders among health care workers research needs. AAOHN Journal. 2008;**56**:487-494

[8] Garosi E, Mazloumi A, Kalantari R, Vahedi Z, Shirzhiyan Z. Design and ergonomic assessment of an infusion set connector tool used in nursing work. Applied Ergonomics. 2019b;**75**:91-98

[9] Mark G, Smith AP. Occupational stress, job characteristics, coping, and the mental health of nurses. British Journal of Health Psychology. 2012;**17**:505-521

[10] Mealer M, Jones J, Newman J, McFann KK, Rothbaum B, Moss M. The presence of resilience is associated with a healthier psychological profile in intensive care unit (ICU) nurses: Results of a national survey. International Journal of Nursing Studies. 2012;**49**:292-299

[11] Carayon P, Karsh B-T, Gurses AP, Holden RJ, Hoonakker P, Schoofs Hundt A, et al. Macroergonomics in health care quality and patient safety. Reviews of Human Factors and Ergonomics. 2013;**8**:4-54

[12] Damanpour F. Organizational complexity and innovation: Developing and testing multiple contingency models. Management Science. 1996;**42**:693-716

[13] Lestari SA, Ginting R. Macro Ergonomic Analysis and Design for Optimizing the Work Environment: A Literature Review. Jurnal Sistem Teknik Industri. 28 Jan 2023;**25**(1):56-64

[14] Hendrick HW, Kleiner B. Macroergonomics: Theory, Methods, and Applications. Boca Raton: CRC Press; 2016

[15] Danesh MK, Garosi E, Mazloumi A, Najafi S. Identifying factors influencing cardiac care nurses' work ability within the framework of the SEIPS model. Work (Reading, Mass.). 2020;**66**(3):569-577. DOI: 10.3233/wor-203199. PMID: 32623418

[16] Punnett L, Warren N, Henning R, Nobrega S, Cherniack M, Team C-NR. Participatory ergonomics as a model

for integrated programs to prevent chronic disease. Journal of Occupational and Environmental Medicine. 2013;**55**:S19-S24

[17] Guimarães LDM, Ribeiro J, Renner J, De Oliveira P. Worker evaluation of a macroergonomic intervention in a Brazilian footwear company. Applied Ergonomics. 2014;**45**:923-935

[18] Adelt F, Weyer J, Fink RD. Governance of complex systems: Results of a sociological simulation experiment. Ergonomics. 2014;**57**:434-448

[19] Murphy LA, Robertson MM, Carayon P. The next generation of macroergonomics: Integrating safety climate. Accident; Analysis and Prevention. 2014;**68**:16-24

[20] Clack L, Kuster SP, Giger H, Giuliani F, Sax H. Low-hanging fruit for human factors design in infection prevention—Still too high to reach? American Journal of Infection Control. 2014;**42**:679-681

[21] Karsh B-T, Waterson P, Holden RJ. Crossing levels in systems ergonomics: A framework to support 'mesoergonomic'inquiry. Applied Ergonomics. 2014;**45**:45-54

[22] Carayon P, Wetterneck TB, Rivera-Rodriguez AJ, Hundt AS, Hoonakker P, Holden R, et al. Human factors systems approach to healthcare quality and patient safety. Applied Ergonomics. 2014;**45**:14-25

[23] Village J, Searcy C, Salustri F, Patrick Neumann W. Design for human factors (DfHF): A grounded theory for integrating human factors into production design processes. Ergonomics. 2015;**58**:1529-1546

[24] Waterson P, Robertson MM, Cooke NJ, Militello L, Roth E, Stanton NA. Defining the methodological challenges and opportunities for an effective science of sociotechnical systems and safety. Ergonomics. 2015;**58**:565-599

[25] Salas E, Grossman R, Hughes AM, Coultas CW. Measuring team cohesion: Observations from the science. Human Factors. 2015;**57**:365-374

[26] Kleiner BM, Hettinger LJ, DeJoy DM, Huang Y-H, Love PE. Sociotechnical attributes of safe and unsafe work systems. Ergonomics. 2015;**58**:635-649

[27] RealyvásquezA,Maldonado-MacíasAA, García-Alcaraz J, Cortés-Robles G, Blanco-Fernández J. Structural model for the effects of environmental elements on the psychological characteristics and performance of the employees of manufacturing systems. International Journal of Environmental Research and Public Health. 2016;**13**:104

[28] Bolis I, Sznelwar LI. A case study of the implementation of an ergonomics improvement committee in a Brazilian hospital–challenges and benefits. Applied Ergonomics. 2016;**53**:181-189

[29] Steege LM, Dykstra JG. A macroergonomic perspective on fatigue and coping in the hospital nurse work system. Applied Ergonomics. 2016;**54**:19-26

[30] Azadeh A, Haghighi SM, Gaeini Z, Shabanpour N. Optimization of healthcare supply chain in context of macro-ergonomics factors by a unique mathematical programming approach. Applied Ergonomics. 2016;**55**:46-55

[31] Yang Y, Asan O. Designing patient-facing health information technologies for the outpatient settings: A literature review. Journal of innovation in health informatics. 2016;**23**:441-449

[32] Meshkati N, Tabibzadeh M, Farshid A, Rahimi M, Alhanaee G.

People-technology-ecosystemintegration: A framework to ensure regional interoperability for safety, sustainability, and resilience of interdependent energy, water, and seafood sources in the (Persian) gulf. Human Factors. 2016;**58**:43-57

[33] Thatcher A, Yeow PH. A sustainable system of systems approach: A new HFE paradigm. Ergonomics. 2016;**59**:167-178

[34] Holden RJ, Valdez RS, Schubert CC, Thompson MJ, Hundt AS. Macroergonomic factors in the patient work system: Examining the context of patients with chronic illness. Ergonomics. 2017;**60**:26-43

[35] Coelho DA, Tavares CSD, Lima TM, Lourenço ML. Psychosocial and ergonomic survey of office and field jobs in a utility company. International Journal of Occupational Safety and Ergonomics. Sep 2018;**24**(3):475-486. DOI: 10.1080/10803548.2017.1331620. Epub 2017 Aug 4. PMID: 28589755

[36] Murphy LA, Robertson MM, Huang Y-H, Jeffries S, Dainoff MJ. A sociotechnical systems approach to enhance safety climate in the trucking industry: Development of a methodology. Applied Ergonomics. 2018b;**66**:82-88

[37] Murphy LA, Huang Y-H, Robertson MM, Jeffries S, Dainoff MJ. A sociotechnical systems approach to enhance safety climate in the trucking industry: Results of an in-depth investigation. Applied Ergonomics. 2018a;**66**:70-81

[38] Thatcher A, Waterson P, Todd A, Moray N. State of science: Ergonomics and global issues. Ergonomics. 2018;**61**:197-213

[39] Carayon P, Hundt AS, Karsh B, Gurses AP, Alvarado C, Smith M, et al. Work system design for patient safety: The SEIPS model. BMJ Quality & Safety. 2006;**15**:i50-i58

[40] Zakerian SA, Garosi E, Abdi Z, Bakhshi E, Kamrani M, Kalantari R. Studying the influence of workplace design on productivity of bank clerks. Journal of Health and Safety at Work. 2016;**6**:35-42

[41] Rostamabadi A, Zamanian Z, Sedaghat Z. Factors associated with work ability index (WAI) among intensive care units'(ICUs') nurses. Journal of Occupational Health. 2017;**59**:147-155

[42] Mohammadi Zeidi E, Farmanbar R, Hoseyni S. Assessment of psychometric properties (validity and reliability) of safety climate questionnaire: Factor analysis application. Journal of Guilan University of Medical Sciences. 2012;**21**:12-21

[43] Kloimüller I, Karazman R, Geissler H, Karazman-Morawetz I, Haupt H. The relation of age, work ability index and stress-inducing factors among bus drivers. International Journal of Industrial Ergonomics. 2000;**25**:497-502

[44] Marqueze EC, Voltz GP, Borges FN, Moreno CR. A 2-year follow-up study of work ability among college educators. Applied Ergonomics. 2008;**39**:640-645

[45] Samadi S, Golmohammadi A. Study the relation between occupational stress and work ability index among nurses of selected military hospital. Journal of Police Medicine. 2013;**2**:223-223

[46] Botha WE, Bridger R. Anthropometric variability, equipment usability and musculoskeletal pain in a group of nurses in the Western cape. Applied Ergonomics. 1998;**29**:481-490

[47] Gharibi V, et al. Effects of work-related stress on work ability index

among Iranian workers. Safety and Health at Work. 2016;**7**(1):43-48

[48] Mazloumi A, Rostamabadi A, Saraji GN, Foroushani AR. Work ability index (WAI) and its association with psychosocial factors in one of the petrochemical industries in Iran. Journal of Occupational Health. 2012;**54**:112-118

[49] Garosi E, Kalantari R, Zanjirani FA, Zuaktafi M, Hosseinzadeh RE, Bakhshi E. Concerns About Verbal Communication in the Operating Room: A Field Study. Human Factors. 2020;**62**(6):940-953. DOI: 10.1177/0018720819858274

[50] Safari S, Akbari J, Kazemi M, Mououdi MA, Mahaki B. Personnel's health surveillance at work: Effect of age, body mass index, and shift work on mental workload and work ability index. Journal of Environmental and Public Health. 2013;**2013**:1-6. Article ID 289498

[51] Steege LM, Pasupathy KS, Drake DA. A work systems analysis approach to understanding fatigue in hospital nurses. Ergonomics. 2018;**61**:148-161

[52] Heyam DF, Besher G, Nesreen A-K. Work ability index of shift working hospital nurses in Jordan. The open nursing journal. 2018;**12**:116